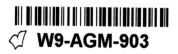

Integrating Complementary Health Procedures into Practice

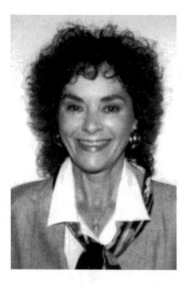**Carolyn Chambers Clark**, EdD, RN, ARNP, FAAN, HNC, is on the Doctoral Faculty at Walden University, and on the graduate health promotion faculty at Schiller International University. Dr. Clark is Founder, the Wellness Institute, and Founding Editor, *Alternative Health Practitioner: The Journal of Complementary and Natural Care.* Her book, *Wellness Practitioner: Concepts, Research, and Strategies, 2nd Edition* (Springer, 1996), won an American Journal of Nursing Book-of-the-Year Award. She has published widely on complementary health topics and is Editor-in-Chief of *Encyclopedia of Complementary Health Practice* (Springer, 1999). Dr. Clark is certified as an holistic practitioner by the American Holistic Nurses Association and has been a member of the American Academy of Nursing since 1980. She serves as a research grant reviewer for Sigma Theta Tau International.

Integrating Complementary Health Procedures into Practice

Carolyn Chambers Clark
EdD, RN, ARNP, HNC, FAAN

 Springer Publishing Company

Copyright © 2000 by Carolyn Chambers Clark

Springer Publishing Company, Inc.
536 Broadway
New York, NY 10012-3955

Acquisitions Editors: Ruth Chasek, Sheri W. Sussman
Production Editor: J. Hurkin-Torres
Cover design by James Scotto-Lavino

99 00 01 02 03 / 5 4 3 2 1

Library of Congress Cataloging-in-Publication Data

Integrating complementary health procedures into practice / Carolyn Chambers Clark
    p. cm.
  Includes bibliographical references and index.
  ISBN 0-8261-1288-9 (hardcover)
  1. Alternative medicine. I. Clark, Carolyn Chambers. II. Encyclopedia of complementary health practice. III. Title: Integrating complementary health procedures into practice.
  [DNLM: 1. Alternative Medicine. 2. Professional Practice. WB 890 I606 1999
R733.I575 1999
615.5—dc21
DNLM/DLC
for Library of Congress   99-28875
                                            CIP

Printed in the United States of America

Any medical, health, or therapeutic agent or procedure described in this book should be applied by the practitioner under appropriate supervision in accordance with professional standards of care and the unique circumstances of each situation.

CONTENTS

C. Mind/Body Approaches

D. Therapeutic Activities

LIST OF TABLES

LIST OF ILLUSTRATIONS

Figures

PREFACE

Integrating Complementary Health Procedures Into Practice is meant to provide health care practitioners with specific ways to integrate complementary health procedures into their practice. This volume is also meant for health care practitioners who wish to be informed about complementary practices for the purpose of making client referrals to complementary practitioners or monitoring their client's complementary treatment.

The term patient is used throughout when referring to allopathic practice because in that world view, the consumer is more passive and is expected to bow to the decisions of the expert practitioner. The term client or health care consumer is used when referring to complementary practice because in that world view, the client is actively engaged in planning for and participating in his or her wellness or well-being. For more about world views, see Chapter 2.

Having been educated as both an allopathic and a complementary practitioner, I believe I am able to identify the strengths and limitations of each, and am knowledgeable about how to integrate the two. Over the past twenty years, I have been studying (often through apprenticeships), trying out, and researching which complementary procedures are effective with which individuals. Two experiences have added tremendously to my knowledge base: as editor of *Alternative Health Practitioner: The Journal of Complementary and Natural Care* since 1995, and editor-in-chief of *The Encyclopedia of Complementary Health Practice*.

This book can be used alone or as a companion volume to *The Encyclopedia of Complementary Health Practices* (Springer Publishing Company, 1999), which provides the theory, history, research base for practice, legal aspects, and uses for complementary practices. *Integrating Complementary Health Procedures Into Practice* is primarily a how-to volume. Together they provide the depth and breadth of information needed by practitioners. Because health care seekers often visit complementary practitioners, allopathic health care practitioners should stay informed of the burgeoning field of complementary practice in order to perform accurate assessments, devise effective treatment plans, incorporate complementary procedures into their practice, communicate with their complementary counterparts, and make referrals to complementary practitioners as needed.

The first section of the book deals with general principles of integration. This includes reasons for integrating complementary procedures into practice, ways of overcoming resistance with clients and other health professionals, scientific support for complementary procedures, elements of the practitioner/client relationship in complementary therapies, choosing the right therapy for the condition at hand, evaluating results, costs, and insurance coverage for complementary procedures.

The second section of this book focuses on the actual complementary procedures. I have included only those I have used both personally and professionally with success: Ayurveda, art production/ritual, Chinese health and healing, Feng Shui, guided imagery, herbs, hypnosis, journalling, meditation, nutrition/supplements, relaxation therapy, sound/music therapy, and touch.

Each practice is organized as follows: detailed definitions and explanatory concepts, directions for use, cautions, application of use (including case studies, clinical forms for assessment, treatment, and referral).

A final resources section provides additional training programs in complementary health care procedures. Organizations and certifying bodies for the various practices are also listed there.

I wish you well on your journey toward integration. Remember, this is a new enterprise and nothing is set in stone. Give yourself time, patience, and nurturance.

Yours in Wellness,

Carolyn Chambers Clark

Carolyn Chambers Clark, RN, ARNP, EdD, FAAN, HNC

PART I
GENERAL PRINCIPLES

1

REASONS FOR INTEGRATING COMPLEMENTARY HEALTH PROCEDURES INTO PRACTICE

There are numerous reasons to integrate complementary procedures into practice. Some of the most important are: failures of the allopathic system of health care, resurgence of old diseases, the impact of a changing environment, consumer interest in complementary procedures, health care provider interest in complementary care, enhanced communication, reduction in health care costs, less invasive procedures with fewer side effects, more attention to the uniqueness of individuals, wellness as a focus, and the self-healing properties of individuals.

FAILURES OF THE ALLOPATHIC SYSTEM OF HEALTH CARE

The conceptual approach of an *allopathic system of health care* affects how health care consumers are viewed. The focus is on disease and the physical body. Patients are viewed as relatively passive in the diagnosis and treatment phases and are believed to react similarly to invaders (viruses, bacteria, etc.) that cause disease. The major function of the practitioner is to distinguish among invaders and remove, destroy, or immobilize them, thus affecting a cure.

Allopathic approaches may be of great value in many acute or emergency situations, although complementary procedures may also be helpful. Complementary procedures are excellent for the chronic conditions that now plague Americans (Micozzi, 1996). One explanation that has been given for both the allopathic conceptualization of treatment and its failure is that United States physicians learn their science by examining dead bodies or cadavers. This study of dead tissue to understand living, breathing humans and the quest for a "magic bullet" to cure all ills is based on a materialistic and reductionistic view of treatment that may not match living, breathing humans (Micozzi, 1996; Cassidy, 1996).

Many times, there is no "magic bullet" cure. A holistic approach is consistent with the complex nature of human beings. A lifestyle change and a multifaceted approach may be necessary.

Other problems with an allopathic approach include: it is frequently rushed; and it often negates the personal, spiritual, and unique experience of clients as well as the importance of client participation in treatment and its evaluation (Micozzi, 1996; Cassidy, 1996).

Another major problem with allopathic approaches is the misuse or overuse of antibiotics (Mainous, Hueston, & Love, 1998). Individuals with cold symptoms may either demand or be given bacteria-treating medications when they have no effect on viruses, making them unnecessary and damaging to the body's naturally occurring bacteria. As bacteria become resistant to more and more antibiotics, eventually there will be no way to treat them.

Additionally, evidence is accumulating rapidly that complementary procedures often are as effective or more effective than allopathic treatments of identical conditions. Complementary approaches may even provide more valuable effects when combined with allopathic approaches (Benor, 1993; Byrd, 1988; Jacobs, Jimenez, & Gloyd, 1994; Jobst, 1995; O'Connor, 1995).

RESURGENCE OF OLD DISEASES

Although allopathy has made some inroads against chronic and degenerative disease, overall their impact is growing. Twenty-five percent of the population has some form of heart or circulatory disease, making it the leading cause of death. However, if trends continue, cancer will surpass heart disease as the leading cause of death and the prevalence of chronic lung disease, hepatitis B, tuberculosis, Alzheimer's disease, end-stage renal disease, diabetes, Lyme disease, chronic fatigue syndrome, chronic migraine headaches, and environmentally caused illness is on the increase (Collinge, 1996).

With this kind of challenge, all available treatment options must be considered. Complementary approaches are coming of age and offer an unprecedented opportunity for enhancing allopathic treatment.

THE IMPACT OF A CHANGING ENVIRONMENT

Recent changes in the environment present new challenges to remaining healthy and well. Crowding and urbanization brings a growing segment of the population into contact with intelligent viruses, bacteria, and pathogens capable of evolving faster than new drugs can be developed to treat them. These changes call out for enhanced preventive and primary care practitioners to treat increasing numbers of individuals exposed to opportunistic diseases who show a compromised resistance to them. An increase in international commerce and immigration contributes to the number and diversity of pathogens our immune systems must conquer. As the population grows and expands into animal habitats, cross-species transfer of pathogens is increased. With the growth in international travel and the movement of military personnel into new environments and then back into the United States, new pathogens are introduced into the general population (Collinge, 1996).

An advantage of some complementary methods is that they strengthen the immune system and promote general well-being. For example, some herbs such as echinacea and astragalus are immune system enhancers, and hypnosis (De-Beneditts, Cigada, & Bianchi, 1994) has been shown to work via brain-immune pathways.

CONSUMER INTEREST IN COMPLEMENTARY PROCEDURES

Eisenberg and colleagues' (1993) groundbreaking study provided evidence that consumers are very interested in complementary procedures. Americans made 425 million visits to complementary practitioners in 1990, exceeding the number of visits to primary care physicians (388 million). This is impressive, considering that many of the treatments are not covered by insurance and clients were forced to pay for care themselves ($10.3 billion as compared to hospitalizations of $12.8 billion).

Eisenberg and colleagues (1993) also found that a large number of individuals do not tell their allopathic practitioner that they are also using complementary treatments. In essence, both allopathic and complementary practitioners are working in the dark with these consumers of health care, unaware of a large part of what might be influencing treatment outcomes. By offering complementary procedures health care practitioners will be privy to a larger percentage, if not the whole, amount of treatment obtained.

Users of complementary procedures are, on the whole, satisfied with the results of their treatment (Emad, 1994; Hare, 1993; O'Connor, 1995). Who are the primary users of these procedures? Surveys indicate they are mainly urban, female and well-educated with middle to high incomes (Cassileth, Lusk, Strouse, & Budenheimer, 1984; Eisenberg et al., 1993; McGuire, 1994). This is a population not easily misled and one well able to judge the quality of care received.

Other characteristics of seekers of complementary procedures have been identified by Cassidy (1996). Such individuals have a high need for affiliation and want a relationship with their practitioner; they wish to alleviate symptoms gradually with fewer side effects; they want the spiritual and emotional aspects of their personhood addressed, are concerned about the invasiveness of typical medical procedures, want to prevent disease and enhance wellness, and/or refuse to take "hopeless" or "terminal" for a diagnosis.

HEALTH CARE PROVIDER INTEREST
IN COMPLEMENTARY CARE

A 1994 survey of allopathic physicians from diverse specialties found that more than 60% were already recommending complementary therapies to their patients. Forty-seven percent reported using complementary therapies themselves and 23% integrated them into their practices (Borkan, Neher, Anson, & Smoker, 1994).

A survey of 300 family physicians in New England found 90% considered complementary therapies legitimate. Indeed, most of the respondents desired training in complementary therapies themselves (Berman et al., 1995).

Medical schools across the country are offering survey courses in the history and philosophy of complementary procedures (Daly, 1997). Some schools of medicine already offering complementary courses are listed in Table 1.1.

Continuing medical education credit has not yet been granted for some courses, but the possibility is being debated (Frieden, 1997), while others are elective or even required courses in the school of medicine (Moore, 1998).

ENHANCED COMMUNICATION

Like any system, the nation's health care system can be improved. The most common complaint consumers have is that they feel their physician does not really listen to them. When clients attempt to explain what is wrong or what they need, allopaths have been trained to cut off such communication, preferring to make their own diagnosis and treatment plan (Koop, 1996).

It may be that one of the reasons consumers are drawn to complementary practices is that they frequently allow free communication between client and practitioner. Complementary practitioners tend to use themselves as part of the treatment. The relationship between practitioner and client is often as important as more tangible treatments. Such practice is validated by mental health constructs, e.g., under stress, humans often need and respond positively to the support of being understood and valued. Complementary systems offer a paradigm for providing this much needed supportive experience. See Chapter 4 for more on this process.

REDUCTION IN HEALTH CARE COSTS

Most complementary practices are much less expensive than the MRIs and surgery of allopathic medicine. When complementary practices are combined with allopathic treatment, interesting results are found. For example, insurance statistics in France (L'Association Francaise d'Acupuncture, 1993) showed that physicians who also practiced acupuncture at least half-time use considerably fewer laboratory examinations, hospitalizations, and prescriptions for medication. (For more information on costs of complementary treatments, see Chapter 7.)

Table 1.1 Schools of Medicine Offering Complementary Health Courses

State	Medical School
Arizona	University of Arizona, Tucson
California	Stanford University, Palo Alto
	University of California, Irvine
	University of California, Los Angeles
	University of California, San Diego
	University of California, San Francisco
Colorado	University of Colorado, Denver
District of Columbia	Georgetown University
	Howard University
Florida	University of Florida, Gainesville
Georgia	Emory University
Illinois	Finch University of Health Sciences/Chicago Medical School, Chicago
	Southern Illinois University, Springfield
Indiana	Indiana University
Kansas	University of Kansas
Kentucky	University of Louisville
Maryland	John Hopkins University
	University of Maryland
Massachusetts	Boston University
	Harvard
Michigan	University of Michigan
	Mayo Medical School
Minnesota	University of Minnesota
Mississippi	University of Mississippi
Missouri	St. Louis University
	Washington University
Nebraska	University of Nebraska
Nevada	University of Nevada
New Hampshire	Dartmouth University
New Jersey	New Jersey Medical School, Newark
	New Jersey Medical School, Piscataway
New Mexico	University of New Mexico
New York	Albany Medical College
	Albert Einstein College
	Columbia University
	Cornell University
	Mount Sinai School of Medicine
	New York Medical College, Valhalla
	State University of New York, Buffalo
	State University of New York, Stony Brook
	State University of New York, Syracuse
North Carolina	Duke University

(continued)

Table 1.1   *(continued)*

State	Medical School
Ohio	Ohio State University
Pennsylvania	Allegheny University of Health Sciences
	Pennsylvania State University, Hershey
	University of Pennsylvania
	University of Pittsburgh
Rhode Island	Brown University
South Carolina	University of South Carolina
Texas	University of Texas, Houston
Utah	University of Utah
Vermont	University of Vermont College
Virginia	Eastern Virginia Medical School, Norfolk
	University of Virginia, Charlottesville
West Virginia	Marshall University
	West Virginia University, Morgantown
Wisconsin	University of Wisconsin, Madison

LESS INVASIVE PROCEDURES WITH FEWER SIDE EFFECTS

Allopathic treatments are often more invasive and have more painful and some-times disastrous side effects than complementary procedures. An estimated 140,000 Americans die every year from adverse prescription drug reactions (Classen, 1997) as compared to 46,000 a year from breast cancer and 40,000 a year from AIDS. Nearly 30% of hospital admissions are due to prescription drug-related problems (Johnson, 1996; Nelson, 1996). Many prescribed drugs have never been tested for their side effects except in short-term studies conducted by the drug companies manufacturing the product. As a result, long-term users may have side effects not found in the research studies.

Another problem with allopathic medications is that many individuals take multiple prescribed drugs; the results of these drug interactions is unknown (because they have never been tested), except by the individual who ingests them. Those individuals are often unable to discern what negative reaction is due to which drug (Mindell & Hopkins, 1998).

Although the public may believe allopathic procedures have been well-re-searched, studies reveal that only 30% of allopathic treatments have been tested adequately (Andersen, 1990; Altman, 1994). Another problem with allopathic treatments is that approximately 20% of illnesses that lead to hospitalization are iatrogenic, that is, caused by allopathic care itself (Greenwood & Nunn, 1994).

Additionally, many prescription drugs have a negative effect on nutrition absorption (Tschanz, 1996). Some decrease appetite and are of concern for populations already at risk nutritionally, including the elderly, those with a chronic disease, dieters, those who abuse alcohol, cigarette smokers, new mothers, adolescents, and certain ethnic minorities (Clark, 1996).

THE UNIQUENESS OF INDIVIDUALS

As any experienced practitioner knows, individuals are unique. This holds true whether working in an allopathic or complementary framework. If it were not the case, allopaths would not have to try more than one medication or dosage with their patients in order to obtain a desired effect. Still, a basic tenet of allopathic practice is that all individuals are basically the same and therefore treatments for a diagnosis are identical (Watkins, 1996).

Age, personality, education, history, gender, geography, employment, and countless other variables blend together and a unique individual in a unique time and place emerges. Practitioners who wish to be most effective and helpful take these factors into account.

WELLNESS AS A FOCUS

Wellness differs from health. It is not merely a state conferred upon others by health care professionals. Clients are experts in evaluating their own well-being. Wellness engages clients in active participation to find a balanced state that is right for them and addresses their physical body, mental, emotional, spiritual, environmental, and interpersonal needs (Clark, 1996), while allopathic practice views a patient as passive and focuses only on the physical body (Watkins, 1996).

In complementary approaches, there is no one dose that is right for all. Situations, unique views, history, and many other factors are examined and contribute to finding the appropriate treatment. Balance, not cure, is the goal.

THE SELF-HEALING PROPERTIES OF INDIVIDUALS

Despite the wish for a "magic bullet" that can undo various negative experiences individuals either choose or are placed in, there probably is no such thing. Instead of searching for a magic pill, complementary practitioners opt to support the innate healing capabilities of the human body, focusing on the body's own ability to heal itself after injury or surgery. A cut, scratch, or virus alerts the body's immune system and it quickly goes to work, as long as the immune system is healthy. Many complementary procedures help strengthen, or assist the client to eliminate factors that are weakening, their immune system.

COMBINING ALLOPATHIC AND COMPLEMENTARY APPROACHES

For the reasons described above, it behooves allopathic practitioners to integrate complementary procedures into their practice. Although they seem drastically different in philosophy, theory and approach, there is much in common.

One of the myths held by some allopaths is that unqualified and unlicensed individuals practice complementary methods. However, the majority of those providing such treatment are allopathically educated (Cassileth, Lusk, Strouse, & Bodenheimer, 1984).

Practitioners educated in both approaches are uniquely qualified to recognize the limitations of both systems. They are able to decide which therapeutic approach will likely be most effective, based on the needs of the client (Watkins, 1996).

A model for such practice has existed since the early 1980s in England when the British Holistic Medical Association (BHMA) was formed. In experimental health centers, such as one situated in the crypt of a London church, allopathic and complementary approaches have been integrated. The primary care physician has initial contact with the client, involving complementary practitioners as appropriate. Both types of practitioners meet to discuss individual clients to ensure that physical, mental, emotional, and spiritual needs are met (Watkins, 1996).

It can be argued that both allopathic and complementary approaches are reductionistic to some extent. Although allopaths do diagnose and often treat all individuals who have the same diagnosis similarly, there is leeway to call in mental health consultants who often deal with emotional aspects of the problem. Additionally, hospitals have chaplains to assist clients with the spiritual aspects of their condition. So, allopaths are not completely reductionistic in their approach.

Likewise, complementary practitioners must reduce their treatment to general principles, else how would the acupuncturist know where to place acupuncture needles, or the aromatherapist know which essential oils to use, or even the therapeutic touch practitioner know how to assess energy fields? (See Chapter 3 for examples of how allopaths also use energy field concepts.)

From this discussion, it is possible to conclude that both systems, allopathic and complementary, have much in common. Their philosophical stances are not as different as generally supposed. Hopefully, political, economic, and personal prejudices on the part of both types of practitioners can be overcome so that integration can occur.

REFERENCES

Altman D. (1994). The scandal of poor medical research. *Brit Med J* 308:283–284.

Andersen B. (1990). *Methodological Errors in Medical Research.* Oxford: Blackwell Scientific Publications.

Benor D. (1993). *Healing Research: Holistic Energy Medicine and Spirituality.* Munich: Helix Verlag.

Berman M, Krishna Singh B, Lao L, Singh BB, Ferentz KS, & Hartnolls SM. (1995). Physicians' attitudes toward complementary or alternative medicine: A regional survey. *Alternative Medicine* 8:361–366.

Borkan J, Neher JO, Anson O, & Smoker B. (1994). Referrals for alternative therapies. *Journal of Family Practice* 39:545–550.

Byrd RC. (1988). Positive therapeutic effects of intercessory prayer in a coronary care unit population. *South Med J* 81:826–829.

Cassidy CM. (1996). Cultural context of complementary and alternative medicine systems. In MS Micozzi (Ed.), *Fundamentals of Complementary and Alternative Medicine* (pp. 9–34). New York: Churchill Livingstone.

Cassileth B, Lusk E, Strouse R, & Bodenheimer B. (1984). Contemporary unorthodox treatments in cancer medicine, a study of patients, treatments and practitioners. *Ann Intern Med* 101:105–112.

Clark CC. (1996). *Wellness Practitioner: Concepts, Research, and Strategies.* New York: Springer Publishing Co.

Classen D. (1997). Adverse drug events in hospitalized patients. *JAMA* 277:301–306.

Collinge W. (1996). *The American Holistic Health Association Complete Guide to Alternative Medicine.* New York: Time Warner.

Daly DS. (1997). Alternative medicine courses taught at United States medical schools: An ongoing listing. *J Altern Comple Med* 3(2):195–197.

Frieden J. (1997). Some family practitioners are using alternative medicine. *Family Practice News* May 1:51.

DeBeneditts G, Cigada M, & Bianchi A. (1994). Autonomic changes during hypnosis: A heart rate variability power spectrum analysis as a marker of sympatho-vagal imbalance. *Int J Clin Exp Hypnosis* 42(2):140–152.

Eisenberg D, Kessler R, Foster C, Norlock F, Culkins D, & Delbanco R. (1993). Unconventional medicine in the United States: Prevalence, costs and patterns of use. *N Engl J Med* 328:246–252.

Emad M. (1994). Does acupuncture hurt? Ethnographic evidence of shifts in psychobiological experiences in pain. *Proc Soc Acupunct Res* 2:129–140.

Greenwood M, & Nunn P. (1994). *Paradox and Healing, Medicine, Mythology and Transformation.* 3rd edition. Victoria, British Columbia: Paradox Publ.

Hare M. (1993). The emergence of an urban U.S. Chinese medicine. *Med Anthropol* 7:30–49.

Jacobs J, Jimenez LM, & Gloyd SS. (1994). Treatment of acute childhood diarrhea with homeopathic medicine: A randomized clinical trial in Nicaragua. *Pediatrics* 93(5):719–725.

Jobst KA. (1995). A critical analysis of acupuncture in pulmonary disease: Efficacy and safety of the acupuncture needle. *J Altern Comple Med* 1:57–85.

Johnson J. (1996). Drug related morbidity and mortality—a cost of illness model. *Arch Intern Med* October 9:155.

Koop CE. (1996). The art and science of medicine. In MS Micozzi (Ed.), *Fundamentals of Complementary and Alternative Medicine* (pp. ix–xi). New York: Churchill Livingstone.

L'Association Francaise d'Acupuncture. (1993). Paris. Unpublished insurance documents.

Mainous AG, Hueston WJ, & Love MM. (1998). Antibiotics for colds in children. *Archives of Pediatric Adolesc Medicine* 152(4):349–352.

McGuire MB. (1994). *Ritual Healing in Suburban America.* New Brunswick, NJ: Rutgers University Press.

Micozzi MS. (1996). Characteristics of complementary and alternative medicine. In MS Micozzi (Ed.), *Fundamentals of Complementary and Alternative Medicine* (pp. 3–8). New York: Churchill Livingstone.

Mindell E, & Hopkins V. (1998). *Prescription Alternatives.* New Canaan, CT: Keats Publishing Company.

Moore NG. (1998). A review of alternative medicine courses taught at US medical schools. *Alternative Therapies* 4(3):90–101.

Nelson K. (1996). Drug-related hospital admissions. *Pharmacotherapy* 16(4):701–706.

O'Connor BB. (1995). *Healing Traditions, Alternative Medicine and the Health Professions*. Philadelphia: University of Pennsylvania Press.

Tschanz C. (1996). Interactions between drugs and nutrients. *Advances in Pharmacology* 35:6–10.

Watkins AD. (1996). Contemporary context of complementary and alternative medicine. In MS Micozzi (Ed.), *Fundamentals of Complementary and Alternative Medicine* (pp. 49–63). New York: Churchill Livingstone.

2

OVERCOMING RESISTANCE TO COMPLEMENTARY PROCEDURES

Clients and other health care professionals may be resistant to using complementary procedures. This chapter examines sources of resistance and provides suggestions for reducing skepticism.

CULTURAL LEARNING AFFECTS BELIEFS

Although it may be difficult for allopathic thinkers to keep open minds when contemplating therapeutic touch or aromatherapy, a discussion of cultural learning may be of help in dissolving some resistance. History can be an important discussion point. The following points may be helpful for reducing resistance:

> Modern medicine is based on the philosophy of Descarte who believed in rationalism, causality, and objectivity. Allopathic medicine has a world view based on certain assumptions that flow from this philosophy, e.g., that the practitioner is more objective and thus is more expert than the patient; that some diseases are more important, e.g., cancer is more important than asthma; that treatment modalities that cause a change in the physical body are preferred; that physical malfunction, not prevention of physical malfunction, is the focus of treatment; and, nonmaterial explanations of causation are to be rejected. (Cassidy, 1996)

> A different, but just as valid world view is held by many complementary practitioners, e.g., Chinese complementary practitioners. Their world view is based on observations of live clients, not dead cadavers. They developed a way to understand and treat conditions in relationship to their clients and through a detailed assessment process. For them, categories that ignore the uniqueness of each person are useless.

They find the process of what led to an imbalance (be it called depression, weight loss, weight gain, sleeplessness, pain, anxiety or whatever) is more important than forcing a unique individual reaction to fit into a predetermined category. As a result, five clients who complain of depression can receive five different treatment regimes. Although diet, exercise, rest and other physical interventions may be suggested, spiritual and energetic aspects will also be addressed by prescribing yoga, t'ai chi, or moving meditations. Art, dancing and chanting may be prescribed to enhance spiritual/emotional growth. (Cassidy, 1996)

CONCEPTS OF DISEASE AND IMBALANCE

Americans have been brought up with the "world view" of the predominant category of health care in this country, namely, allopathic health care. A hypothetical example can help identify this world view. Pretend that a young woman goes to both an allopathic practitioner and a complementary practitioner complaining of a sore throat. Using allopathic logic, the allopath is apt to identify a *streptococcal bacterium* in the young woman's throat and order an antibiotic.

Using allopathic logic, stop to consider what has just happened. Twenty percent of the population carries that same bacterium in their throats and never develops a sore throat (Greenwood & Nunn, 1994). Also, using Cartesian thinking, consider the fact that bacteria are fast adapting to antibiotics and for some, antibiotics no longer are effective. Additionally, it is important to consider that antibiotics destroy both the bacterium "causing" the sore throat as well as the bacteria in the intestines that help in digestion. By taking the antibiotic and not replacing the "good bacteria" with acidophilus (in yogurt or acidophillus form), digestive side effects are sure to follow.

The complementary practitioner would take a different tack, depending on his or her discipline, but in general, the young woman's unique qualities, her unique history and the unique point in time she chose to come for treatment are all of as much, if not more, importance to diagnosis and treatment. Through discussion and observation, the complementary practitioner might observe that the young woman's voice is very soft and her shoulders are hunched up, very close to her ears. The practitioner might also learn that the young woman is very angry with her mother who told her not to marry the man she loves. Having been raised in a family where expression of feelings, especially negative ones, was not allowed, the young woman's voice becomes louder as she identifies the source of her anger. The complementary practitioner might suggest several treatments and devise a verbal contract with the young woman for the treatments she agrees to work on. For example, the complementary therapist might ask the young woman to write her negative feelings in a private journal, draw her feelings toward her mother, listen daily to a relaxation audiotape with specific hypnotic suggestions about dealing effectively with parents, take a yoga class or engage in stretching exercises to improve posture and release negative feelings, gargle with salt water, increase her intake of vitamin C, and take either the herb astragalus or echinacea to boost her immune system.

THE CONCEPTS OF VITAL ENERGY AND ENERGY FIELDS

Allopathic practitioners work from a physical body-disease model. Many, if not all, complementary practitioners work from a wholeperson energy model. Different complementary disciplines call it by different names—from ch'i to prana—but the idea is the same. Although more ethereal and more difficult to identify, who can say where the physical body, with its ongoing chemical and electrical changes, ends? Does the physical body merge into an energetic body and then into a spiritual body? In addition to working from an energetic conceptual model, most complementary disciplines include the spiritual and emotional components of whole persons in their assessment and treatment.

Allopathic practitioners may find it difficult to accept the concepts of vital energy and energy fields. These frameworks are widely utilized by practitioners of Ayurveda, touch therapies, tai chi, and many other complementary approaches.

One way to deal with resistance to this mind-body-spirit conceptual framework is to point out that allopathic practitioners also attend to body energy and measure it. Different procedures are used, e.g., electrocardiograms (ECGs) and electro-encephalograms.

By identifying how the heart is a primary source of energy in the body, resistance by skeptics can be decreased. Here is a scenario for discussing the importance of energy to allopathic practice.

> The heart's energy can be recorded anywhere on the body. Where does this energy go? Does it stop at the skin's surface? Is it possible that complementary practitioners who work at the energy level are detecting heart and/or brain electrical energy above the skin's surface? (Watkins, 1996)
>
> Remember the last time you walked into a room. Did you feel welcomed or rejected? Did you feel comfortable or uncomfortable? It could be that the atmosphere or "vibes" that you detected when entering that room were actually the electrical energy emanating from the heart or maybe the brain of the individuals present.
>
> Modern digital processing computers have revealed there are three basic types or patterns of heart energy. Research with these computers reflect the activity in the (autonomic) nervous system (Ori, Monir, & Weiss, 1992; Stein, Bosner, Kleiger, & Conger, 1994; McCraty, Atkinson, Tiller, & Watkins, 1995). From these findings, it can be concluded that activity or energy in the nervous system is directly related to heart energy (Watkins, 1996). Negative emotions such as anger and stressful situations increase the energy in the sympathetic nervous system (Kamada, Shinji, & Kumashiro, 1992; Sloan, Shapiro, & Bagiella, 1994). Compassion and caring increase the energy in the parasympathetic nervous system (McCraty et al., 1995). It is also clear that the central nervous system and the immune system function as an integrated whole to maintain a healthy balance in the body (Watkins, 1996). The immune system and brain talk to each other via a complicated system of chemical signals.

Allopaths often are faced with the concept of lack of energy when treating chronic fatigue syndrome, fibromyalgia, depression, and other energy-based conditions. Searches for measurable pathology and the diagnoses of anemia, cancer, and thyroid dysfunction usually are deadend efforts. Lack of energy may be attributed to viral causation by frustrated allopaths when no specific findings appear (Watkins, 1996). Suppose such clients were referred to complementary therapists who practice therapeutic touch, tai chi, or acupressure, measures that may rebalance energy?

PSYCHONEUROIMMUNOLOGY DEMONSTRATES HOW THE BODY AND MIND INTERACT

Allopathic thinkers may also have a difficult time accepting that the mind influences the body and vice versa. Often, mental health professionals and medical-surgical practitioners view each other with suspicion. The relatively new concept of psychoneuroimmunology provides a bridging conceptual framework for reducing this resistance.

Overwhelming evidence has been provided that the brain is capable of regulating all aspects of the immune system (Reichlin, 1993; Blalock, 1994). Thoughts, feelings, and perceptions do alter immunity. It is possible that complementary approaches alter feelings of well-being by activating brain-immune pathways (Watkins, 1996).

Expectation of getting better can also affect the immune system. For example, research has shown that hypnosis can influence brain-immune pathways in some individuals (Neild & Cameron, 1985; DeBeneditts, Cigada, & Bianchi, 1994). See Chapter 3 for scientific support to decrease resistance.

IDENTIFYING RESISTANCE TO CHANGE

Integrating complementary procedures into practice requires change. Resistance to change occurs because something is new and unfamiliar. If integrating complementary skills into practice is viewed as a threat to current status, existing ways of living, job, money, familiar habits, autonomy or free will, resistance to change can be expected. When deciding to integrate complementary procedures into practice, ask the following questions:

1. What other factors will be affected as a result of changing?
2. What forces are operating to inhibit change at this time?
3. What information or experience must precede the change?
4. What new procedures or experiences will need to be developed as a result of the change?
5. Who is likely to be affected by the change?
6. Are all involved aware of the need for change and its purpose?
7. Are all involved sufficiently engaged in planning for the change?
8. What past experiences of those involved might be influencing resistance to change now?

9. How open to change have those involved been to the introduction of change in the past?

IDENTIFYING CLIENT READINESS FOR CHANGE

The Health Belief Model is the best developed model for assessing readiness for change. It is used to predict the likelihood that individuals will change their behavior in order to avoid illness. A factor to assess when identifying client readiness for change is the level of dissatisfaction with current lifestyle.

Table 2.1 provides a format for assessing client readiness for change and current complementary and allopathic treatments already in place. The form can be filled out in the waiting room prior to the first visit and can be used later in treatment to see if resistance to one or more approaches has decreased.

Table 2.1   Use of Complementary and Allopathic Treatments

DIRECTIONS: Read the statements below and circle the number that resembles the importance of each statement to your health and wellness.

Affirmations

1. I already use affirmations to enhance my health and healing.
2. I would like to learn to use affirmations.
3. I have no interest in using affirmations.

Aromatherapy

1. I already use essential oils to enhance my health and healing.
2. I would like to learn to use essential oils.
3. I have no interest in using essential oils.

Ayurveda

1. I am currently using an ayurveda meal plan and herbs to enhance my well-being.
2. I want to learn more about Ayurveda methods of healing.
3. I have no interest in using Ayurveda.

Art/Ritual

1. I use drawings and/or rituals to enhance my healing.
2. I want to learn more about using art and rituals.
3. I have no interest in learning about using art and rituals.

(continued)

Table 2.1   *(continued)*

Breathing Therapy

1. I use breathing techniques to enhance my healing.
2. I want to learn more about using breathing techniques.
3. I have no interest in learning about using breathing techniques.

Chinese Healing

1. I use Chinese healing methods to enhance my healing.
2. I want to learn more about using Chinese healing methods.
3. I have no interest in learning about Chinese healing methods.

Coping Skills Training

1. I use coping skills methods to enhance my healing.
2. I want to learn more about using coping skills methods.
3. I have no interest in learning about coping skills training.

Exercise

1. I use movement and exercise to enhance my healing.
2. I want to learn more about using exercise and movement methods.
3. I have no interest in learning about exercise and movement methods.

Feng Shui

1. I use Feng Shui principles to enhance my healing.
2. I want to learn more about using Feng Shui principles.
3. I have no interest in learning about Feng Shui methods.

Guided Imagery

1. I use guided imagery to enhance my health and healing.
2. I would like to learn more about using guided imagery.
3. I have no interest in learning about guided imagery.

Herbs

1. I use herbs to enhance my health and healing.
2. I want to learn to use herbs.
3. I have no interest in learning to use herbs.

Hypnosis

1. I already use self-hypnosis to enhance my health and healing.

Table 2.1   *(continued)*

2. I want to learn to use self-hypnosis.
3. I have no interest in learning to use hypnosis.

Journal Writing

1. I already use journal writing to enhance my health and healing.
2. I want to learn to use journal writing.
3. I have no interest in learning to use journal writing.

Lifestyle Change

1. I already have changed my lifestyle to enhance my health and healing.
2. I want to learn about using lifestyle change.
3. I have no interest in changing my lifestyle.

Meditation

1. I already meditate to enhance my health and healing.
2. I want to learn about using meditation.
3. I have no interest in using meditation.

Nutrition/Supplements

1. I already use foods and supplements to enhance my health and healing.
2. I want to learn about using nutrition and supplements.
3. I have no interest in learning about using nutrition and supplements.

Relaxation Therapy

1. I already use relaxation methods to enhance my healing.
2. I want to learn about relaxation therapy.
3. I have no interest in learning about using relaxation therapy.

Refuting Irrational Ideas

1. I already refute irrational ideas to enhance my health.
2. I want to learn about refuting irrational ideas.
3. I have no interest in learning to refute irrational ideas.

Sound/Music Therapy

1. I already use sound and/or music to enhance my health.
2. I want to learn about using sound and music.
3. I have no interest in learning to use sound and music.

(continued)

Table 2.1   *(continued)*

Thought Stopping

1. I already use thought stopping to enhance my healing.
2. I want to learn about using thought stopping.
3. I have no interest in learning thought stopping.

Touch Therapies

1. I already use touch therapies to enhance my healing.
2. I want to learn more about using touch therapies.
3. I have no interest in learning touch therapies.

Drugs and Medications I Am Currently Taking (Please include the dosages and times taken for each)

Surgeries I Have Had (Please write down the date and type of surgery)

Go back and look at what you circled: twos indicate readiness for change, while threes indicate resistance to change.

DECREASING CLIENT RESISTANCE TO CHANGE

There are specific steps that can be taken to reduce resistance to change. Centering and relaxation procedures can be used if anxiety or threat are the source of resistance to change. (See Chapter 23.)

Resistance to change will be decreased if change behavior is rewarded. The first step in rewarding movement toward complementary procedures is to identify the countable behaviors that can be changed. Table 2.2 shows examples of behaviors that can and cannot be counted.

Table 2.2   Examples of Behaviors that Can and Cannot Be Counted

Countable Behaviors	Noncountable Behaviors
practicing relaxation exercises	being motivated
ingesting calcium tablets	being depressed
saying affirmations daily	being angry
rearranging a room using Feng Shui principles	improving communication
using guided imagery to reduce pain	feeling guilty
using coping skills statements	grieving
taking ginseng daily	being noncompliant
writing in a journal every evening	being hostile
	feeling anxious
	feeling happy
	feeling deprived
	mistrusting others

Once the behavior is expressed in countable terms, *baseline data* can be gathered. Data consist of information gathered prior to treatment. At the beginning of treatment, behavior is counted to see how often it occurs and clients are asked what is rewarding to them about the behavior. If unable to answer, universal rewards such as attention, smiles, and praise can be used. Table 2.3 shows reinforcers for one client.

Table 2.3   Reinforcers for One Client

Positive, rewarding reinforcers	Negative, depriving reinforcers
listening to music	doing dishes
reading a "good" book	eating celery and carrots
going dancing	vacuuming
eating out	being nagged

To increase the occurrence of positive, goal-directed behavior, practitioners must provide rewards immediately following the behavior. If that is not possible, a written contract, journal entry, or some other method can be used to indicate a reward is due.

Some desired client behaviors may occur at random or very rarely. In these instances, *shaping* techniques can be used to reward approximations to the goal. For example, telling the client the exact words to say or movements to make and then praising the behavior evoked, can also be effective.

Contracting is another method that can decrease resistance to change. When a client takes the time to write up a specific contract and sign it, the goal becomes more concrete. The contract also serves as a reminder of the agreement to pursue the goal.

The more specific, realistic, appropriate, and attainable the goal, the more likely it will be attained. Table 2.4 provides a written contract between the practitioner and client.

Table 2.4   Practitioner-Client Contract

Treatment Goal: To spend 30 minutes every day completing the back strengthening exercises agreed upon.

I, Edith Bracken, agree to spend 30 minutes every day completing back strengthening exercises agreed upon for 2 weeks, whereupon I will treat myself to the purchase of a relaxing music cd. I understand that if I do not fulfill this contract, the designated reward (cd) will not be purchased.

Signed: _____(Client)

_____ (Complementary Practitioner)

_____ (Date)

This chapter has presented ways to reduce resistance to complementary procedures. Methods for overcoming resistance include: discussing cultural learning and world views, pointing out the importance of energetic system thinking, identifying the relationship between psychoneuroimmunology and body-mind interactions, and identifying resistance to and readiness for change.

REFERENCES

Blalock JE. (1994). The immune system: Our sixth Sense. *Immunology* 2:8–13.

Cassidy CM. (1996). Cultural context of complementary and alternative medicine systems. In MS Micozzi (Ed.), *Fundamentals of Complementary and Alternative Medicine* (pp. 9–34). New York: Churchill Livingstone.

DeBeneditts G, Cigada M, & Bianchi A. (1994). Autonomic changes during hypnosis: A heart rate variability power spectrum analysis as a marker of sympatho-vagal balance. *Int J Clin Exp Hypnosis* 42(2):140–152.

Greenwood M, & Nunn P. (1994). *Paradox and Healing, Medicine, Mythology and Transformation.* 3rd ed. Victoria, B.C.: Paradox Publ.

Kamada T, Shinji S, & Kumashiro M. (1992). Power spectral analysis of heart rate variability in type As and type Bs during mental workload. *Psychosom Med* 54:462–470.

McCraty R, Atkinson M, Tiller WA, & Watkins AD. (1995). The effects of emotions on short-term power spectrum analysis of heart variability. *Am J Cardiol* 76(14):1089–1093.

Neild JE, & Cameron IR. (1985). Bronchoconstriction in response to suggestion: Its prevention by an inhaled anticholinergic agent. *J Immunol* 136:2348–2357.

Ori Z, Monir G, & Weiss J. (1992). Heart rate variability. Frequency domain analysis. *Cardiol Clin* 10(3):499–537.

Reichlin S. (1993). Neuroendocrine-immune interactions. *New England Journal of Medicine* 329(17):1246–1253.

Sloan RP, Shapiro PA, & Bagiella E. (1994). Effect of mental stress throughout the day on cardiac autonomic control. *Biol Psychol* 37:L 89–99.

Stein PK, Bosner MS, Kleiger RE, & Conger BM. (1994). Heart rate variability: A measure of cardiac autonomic tone. *Am Heart Journal* 127(5):1376–1381.

Watkins AD. (1996). Contemporary context of complementary and alternative medicine, integrated mind-body medicine. In MS Micozzi (Ed.), *Fundamentals of Complementary and Alternative Medicine* (pp. 49–63). New York: Churchill Livingstone.

3

SCIENTIFIC SUPPORT FOR COMPLEMENTARY PROCEDURES

THE ROLE OF SCIENCE IN TREATMENT

Although it is believed allopathic medicine is based on science, recent studies show that only 30% of procedures have been tested adequately (Altman, 1994; Andersen, 1990). That means 70% of medical practice is based on observation and experience, just as much as complementary practice.

The difference is that many complementary practices evolved long before the Western philosophy of science and empiricism combined into what is today called the scientific method. Ayurveda, aromatherapy, herbology, Chinese health and healing, and other procedures have thousands of years of experience as proof of their efficacy. From their perspective, principles of treatment have been refined and continuously tested through the ages, distilling wisdom gained into effective practice (Collinge, 1996).

Several problems unique to complementary approaches create barriers to research. One problem is that complementary treatments are not aimed at a single pathologic process as are allopaths. Another is that individuals are assumed to be unique, whereas much traditional research is focused on average responses. Allopathic research uses a randomized placebo controlled trial to pinpoint a single treatment's efficacy. Complementary approaches place more emphasis on the individual's validation of treatment effectiveness. For these reasons, designing research with precision and control is difficult, but not impossible (Lewith, 1993).

However, the lack of scientific controls by complementary researchers does not invalidate their findings, it merely makes them less generalizable to other groups of clients. Funding of complementary practices has been primarily limited to small-scale trials that lack statistical significance (Watkins, 1996). Then too, complementary practitioners in this country are not always well-versed in research methods. Additionally, drug companies and others with the resources to study complementary methods are not interested in providing funds for research since there may be no product that can be sold for a profit.

All of these factors explain why complementary research has not burgeoned as allopathic research has. The history of complementary research in this country stands in contrast to the stronger tradition of funding such studies in Europe, especially Great Britain. Nestled in allopathic teaching hospitals, centers of excellence have sprung up. There, well-controlled scientific studies are enhancing clinical decision making. Even there, the focus has been on determining therapeutic efficacy, not on investigating the mechanisms of action of complementary therapies (Watkins, 1996).

One criticism of complementary research is that it is often based on subjective measures of therapeutic benefit. Client perception of change, a reduction of symptoms, or a global sense of enhanced well-being may be dismissed by allopathic practitioners who claim there is no real effect on objective measures of the disease process.

Viewing only quantifiable objective measures as valid overlooks the premise that available tests may not detect the subtle changes occurring during (and after) complementary therapies. Feeling better may be equivalent to being better, despite the fact that objective tests do not substantiate subjective impressions (Watkins, 1996).

Clinical practice is usually guided by the subjective response of clients, not by objective benefits. Individuals do not always perceive objective benefits, but they do know when they feel better. It may be artificial to classify improvement as either subjective or objective when some measures, such as blood pressure, are influenced by subjective factors such as a stressful environment or the interpretation of the clinician. Although a mechanistic, reductionistic approach assumes that subjective and objective results are distinct categories, there is an interaction between the two (Watkins, 1996).

Accumulating psychoneuroimmunology research provides evidence that the immune system and the central nervous system function as an integrated whole. Thoughts, perceptions, and feelings can alter immunity through two mind-body pathways of communication: autonomic and neuroendocrine. Through a rich flow of cytokines, neuropeptides, and hormones, the brain communicates with the immune system. This two-way system confirms that perception affects illness and illness affects perception (Watkins, 1995). It may be that complementary procedures alter subjective feelings of well-being, thereby promoting a healing effect on illness and disease (Watkins, 1994).

FINDING REPORTS OF COMPLEMENTARY
THERAPY RESEARCH

Although there is a great need for more research, positive results from complementary procedures studied are beginning to accumulate. The best place to find these studies is through an internet search using the Medline address: http://

www.nlm.gov/. (There is no charge for an abstract of studies.) The National Center for Complementary and Alternative Medicine can be found at http://altmed.od.nih.gov. The site has information on the center's programs and activities and on advances in the field of complementary medicine.

A SAMPLING OF COMPLEMENTARY RESEARCH FINDINGS

The purpose here is not to provide an in-depth report of research providing support for complementary procedures. For that, consult *The Encyclopedia of Complementary Health Practice*, Springer Publishing Company, 1999. Instead, a sampling of research providing support for various complementary procedures is presented in tabular form.

Table 3.1   The Scientific Validation of Some Herbs

Herbs	Actions	Studies
Garlic	Lowers cholesterol	Sial & Ahmed, 1982
Maharishi Amrit Kalash	Reduces tumor cells	Arnold et al., 1991
Saw Palmetto	Reduces prostate cancer	Champlault, 1984
Urtica Cioica	Reduces rhinitis	Mittman, 1990
Pectin	Lowers glucose levels	Jenkins et al., 1977

Table 3.2   Research Support for Some Other Complementary Procedures

Procedure	Actions	Studies
Ayurveda	Decreased chronic disease symptoms	Janssen, 1989
Breathing therapy	Enhance lung function	Delk et al., 1994
Chinese herbs	Improve survival rates for cancer	Sun, 1988
Hypnosis	Reduce asthmatic symptoms; reduce anxiety	Ewer & Stewart, 1986 Edwards, 1991
Imagery	Increased immune function	Zachariae et al., 1994
(Journal) writing	Increased immune function	Pennebaker et al., 1988
Meditation	Lowered blood pressure; reduce anxiety	Schneider et al., 1991 Kabatt-Zinn et al., 1992
Relaxation therapy	Reduced preventricular contractions; reduced PMS symptoms	Benson et al., 1975 Goodale et al., 1990
Therapeutic touch	Wound healing	Wirth et al., 1993

REFERENCES

Altman D. (1994). The scandal of poor medical research. *Br Med J* 308:283–284.

Andersen B. (1990). *Methodological Errors in Medical Research.* Oxford: Blackwell Scientific Publications.

Arnold J. et al. (1991). Chemopreventive activity of Maharishi Amrit Kalash and related agents in rat tracheal epithelial and human cancer cells. *Proceedings of the Am Assoc for Cancer Research* 32:15–18.

Benson H, Alexander S, & Feldman C. (1975). Decreased premature ventricular contractions through the use of the relaxation response in patients with stable ischemic heart disease. *Lancet* 2:380–382.

Champlault G. (1984). A double-blind trial of an extract of the plant *serenoa repens* in benign prostatic hyperplasia. *Br J Clin Pharmacol* 18:461–462.

Collinge W. (1996). *The American Holistic Health Association Guide to Alternative Medicine.* New York: Time Warner Books.

Delk KK, Geirtz R, Hicks DA, Carden F, & Rucker R. (1994). The effects of biofeedback-assisted breathing retraining on lung function in patients with cystic fibrosis. *Chest* 195(1):23–28.

Edwards D. (1991). A meta-analysis of the effects of meditation and hypnosis on measures of anxiety. *Dissertation Abstracts International* 48(2A):1039.

Ewer TC, & Stewart DE. (1986). Improvement of bronchial hyperresponsiveness in patients with moderate asthma after treatment with a hypnotic technique: A randomised controlled trial. *Br J Med* 293:1129–1132.

Goodale I, Domar A, & Benson H. (1990). Alleviation of premenstrual syndrome symptoms with the relaxation response. *Obstet Gynecol* 75(4):649–655.

Janssen G. (1989). The application of Maharishi Ayur-Veda in the treatment of ten chronic diseases: a pilot study. *NED TIJDSCHR GENEESKD* 5:586–594.

Jenkins DJA, Leeds AR, Gassull, MA, Cochet G, & Alberti KGMM. (1977). Decrease in postprandial insulin and glucose concentrations by guar and pectin. *Ann Intern Med* 86:20–23.

Kabat-Zinn J, Massion A, Kristeller J et al. Effectiveness of a meditation-based stress reduction program in the treatment of anxiety disorders. *Am J Psychiatry* 149(7):936–943.

Lewith T, & Aldridge D. (1993). *Clinical Research Methodology for Complementary Therapies.* London: Hodder and Stoughton.

Mittman, P. (1990). Double-blind randomized study of urtica dioica in treatment of allergic rhinitis. *Planta Medica* 56:44–47.

Pennebaker JW, Kiecolt-Glaser J, & Glaser R. (1988). Disclosure of traumas and immune function: Health implications for psychotherapy. *Journal of Consulting and Clinical Psychology* 56:239–245.

Schneider RH, Staggers F, & Alexander N et al. (1991). Stress management in elderly blacks with hypertension: A preliminary report. *Proceedings of the Second International Conference on Race, Ethnicity and Health: Challenges in Diabetes and Hypertension.* Sponsored by Case Western Reserve University, Salvador Bahia, Brazil.

Sial AY, & Ahmed SI. (1982). Study of the hypotensive action of garlic extract in experimental animals. *Journal of the Pakistan Medical Association* 32(1):237–239.

Sun Y. (1988). The role of traditional Chinese medicine in supportive care of cancer patients. *Recent Results in Cancer Research* 108:327–334.

Watkins AD. (1994). The role of alternative therapy in allergic disease. *Clin Exp Allergy* 24:813–825.

Watkins AD. (1995). Perceptions, emotions and immunity: An integrated homeostatic network. *Q J Med* 88:283–294.

Watkins AD. (1996). Contemporary context of complementary and alternative medicine. In MS Micozzi (Ed.), *Fundamentals of Complementary and Alternative Medicine* (pp. 49–63). New York: Churchill/Livingstone.

Wirth DP, Richardson JT, Eidelman WS, & O'Malley AC. (1993). Full thickness dermal wounds treated with non-contact therapeutic touch: A replication and extension. *Complementary Therapies in Medicine* 1:127–132.

Zachariae R, Hansen JB, Andersen, M, Jinquan T, Petersen KS, Simonsen C, Zachariae C, & Thestrup-Pedersen K. (1994). Changes in cellular immune function after immune specific guided imagery and relaxation in high and low hypnotizable healthy subjects. *Psychotherapy and Psychosomatics* 61(1-2):74–92.

4

THE PRACTITIONER-CLIENT RELATIONSHIP

The original meaning of doctor was teacher, but the word now connotes an allopath who is in charge, and who determines and provides the correct remedy (Collinge, 1996). For many individuals, one of their greatest motives in choosing complementary practitioners is the desire to take greater control over their health. It is suitable, then, that in many complementary approaches, the practitioner takes on the role of teacher or consultant. In these cases, the client is actively involved in enhancing his or her well-being.

For many complementary practitioners, the practitioner-client relationship is viewed as an energy field. The practitioner's emotional and spiritual state is believed to have a direct impact on the client and to have an important influence on the success of treatment. They pray or meditate prior to a session to enhance the practitioner-client energy field.

Other complementary practitioners believe their interventions or approaches are so powerful there is no need to focus on the practitioner-client relationship. This book supports the view that the relationship is key to effective results. It may be the crucial difference between a novice and advanced practitioner (Krieger, 1994).

For many complementary practices, positive benefits accrue in a cumulative manner, whether it is mixing herbs, ingesting specific foods or supplements, using rituals, arranging a health-promoting environment, developing wellness images, saying or thinking positive thoughts, writing in a journal, meditating, using structured relaxation measures, listening to music, or using touch procedures. Taking responsibility for one's health requires time and a reordering of priorities. Many clients may want to participate fully in becoming well, but once they realize how much is involved, some lose interest. It may be necessary for the complementary practitioner to emphasize the potential benefits from such an approach. In addition to improved health, clients can expect an increased level of self-empowerment, enhanced self-esteem, and a sense of pride and accomplishment.

Time is an important variable in the relationship between complementary practitioner and client. It is believed that time must pass in order for the body's self-healing mechanisms to reestablish health. It may be helpful to remind clients of the western cultural preoccupation with speed of recovery. Accustomed to allopathic treatments, they may expect instantaneous results. By reframing the importance of time, clients may be more apt to undertake active involvement in their treatment.

COMMUNICATION SKILLS AND THE PRACTITIONER/ CLIENT RELATIONSHIP

Communication skills are of paramount importance in effective practitioner/client relationships. Listening to what the client says grows in importance when clients expect to have a say in their treatment and to take an active part in feeling better. To enhance client involvement in their treatment, the practitioner takes steps to remove blocks to listening that include: comparing, mind reading, rehearsing, filtering, judging, dreaming, identifying, advising, sparring, being right, derailing, or placating (McKay, Davis, & Fanning, 1995).

Comparing. Often, practitioners only listen partially to clients. This occurs because they are focused on being smarter, more competent, more emotionally healthy, or more put upon.

Mind Reading. Mind reading interferes with paying attention to what the client is saying. During mind reading, the practitioner tries to figure out what the client is really thinking and feeling, rather than listening closely to what is being said.

Rehearsing. During rehearsing, the practitioner is not listening because she is thinking about what to say next. Some people rehearse entire chains of responses, e.g., "If she says that, then I'll say . . . "

Filtering. Sometimes practitioners listen to only part of what is said. Filtering happens most often when the practitioner feels guilty, or threatened, or may not want to hear the client's anger or other negative feeling expressed.

Judging. Judging is one of the most destructive practitioner behaviors. When the client's comments have already been labelled in the practitioner's mind as silly, immaterial, nuts, or unqualified, the possibility of a helpful relationship is greatly reduced.

Dreaming. Something the client says can trigger a chain of private associations in the practitioner. When that happens, active listening ends because the practitioner is paying more attention to his own thoughts than to what the client is saying.

Identifying.   When the practitioner hears what the client says and refers it back to his or her own experience, identifying has occurred. An example of this kind of communication block is when the practitioner thinks about her own pain when the client talks about his.

Advising.   Open communication is hampered when the practitioner does not listen to the full expression of the client's thoughts and feelings. By giving advice before hearing the client's complete statement, the practitioner does not encourage active involvement in treatment.

Sparring.   Sparring occurs when the practitioner disagrees with, discounts, or disparages what the client says. Any or all of these responses block open communication.

Being Right.   Practitioners are often taught in their educational programs that they are the expert. The need to always be right leads to the inability to listen to criticism because mistakes cannot be acknowledged. When the practitioner-client relationship is valued, as it is in many complementary therapies, being the expert practitioner recedes in importance.

Derailing.   Derailing includes changing the subject when bored or uncomfortable, and joking or quipping. All of these conversational behaviors interfere with a therapeutic practitioner-client relationship.

Placating.   The practitioner's ability to show respect and listen actively are important to an effective relationship with clients. Placating, by agreeing with everything the client says just to be pleasant, is detrimental to an honest practitioner-client relationship.

EMPATHY: ACCURATELY PERCEIVING THE CLIENT'S FEELINGS AND MEANINGS

One goal of the practitioner/client relationship is to accurately perceive the client's feelings and meanings. The practitioner does not just become sympathetic, taking on the client's feelings or views. Instead, the practitioner remains separate, trying to understand client views and feelings. For example, the practitioner can be empathic with a crying client without resorting to tears and helplessness. Empathy is a middle state between taking on another's emotions and intellectual objectivity.

When being empathic, the practitioner uses the words and language of the client, reflecting back feelings and ideas (McKay, Davis, & Fanning, 1995), always validating impressions. Empathic communication says: This is what I am hearing, seeing, understanding you to be saying. Am I correct? There is a purposeful action to understand not only the words but also the emotions and body movement being communicated.

ASSERTIVENESS

Helpful complementary practitioners strive to be assertive, neither blaming nor excusing clients who do not follow agreed upon treatment. Client criticism is acknowledged: "Yes, you're right, I am ten minutes late." "You're right, I don't have Sunday hours." Frequent and direct eye contact is made with the client. The practitioner also asks the client for feedback, e.g., "Tell me what you heard me say." Assertive complementary practitioners also teach their clients to be assertive and to value clear, direct communication. (See: Assertiveness, Chapter 16, for more information.)

CENTERING: A METHOD OF ENHANCING THE PRACTITIONER-CLIENT RELATIONSHIP

Centering is a powerful tool for freeing practitioners from becoming too personally identified with client life issues. When practitioners are not centered, they are apt to feel fatigued, stressed, depressed, or angry when working with a client who displays these qualities.

A base of stability is achieved through centering. When the practitioner is centered, communication blocks are reduced and active listening is easier to achieve.

Centering can be achieved while standing or sitting, but to learn the technique, a seated position is often more beneficial. The following directions can be practiced until simply thinking the word, "center," allows the practitioner to achieve a stable, inner stillness.

1. Sit in a comfortable chair with feet flat on the floor and hands resting quietly in the lap.
2. Close the eyes.
3. Check the body for tension spots.
4. On the next inhale, send a wave of relaxation to any identified areas, possibly as a color.
5. On the next exhale, release any tension, perhaps as another color.
6. Continue inhaling and exhaling according to #4 and #5 until feeling relaxed and inwardly still.
7. Gradually, without effort, allow your breathing to move to your center, about the level of your navel.
8. (Optional). Picture the body surrounded by a protective shield that allows positive energy in, but keeps negative energy out. This shield can be conceived as a color, light source, or symbol.

With practice, centering can be achieved quickly. Wellness practitioners have reported the following ways of using centering:

- "I take a moment in my office between clients and get centered."
- "I breathe in a relaxing color as I'm walking down the hall on the way to my next client. When I arrive in the client's room, I feel an inner stillness, an ability to listen and understand whatever he is trying to tell me."
- "I center myself when I'm with a client. I ask her to center herself and we do it together. We both seem to be more relaxed and focused on the treatment that follows when we are both centered."

Clients can be encouraged to center themselves between sessions as a relaxation and focusing method. The steps of centering remain the same. Directions given above can be copied or adapted for use with clients (Clark, 1996).

EVALUATING PRACTITIONER COMMUNICATION SKILLS

Use the information in Table 4.1 to evaluate communication skills with clients and as a guide for devising a plan to improve them.

Table 4.1   Self-Critiquing Practitioner Communication Skills

	Excellent	Average	Needs Practice
During the treatment session, I:			
1. Was prompt.			
2. Was professional.			
3. Answered all client questions.			
4. Listened to all client complaints/comments.			
5. Made comments to the client to indicate I understood his or her concerns.			
6. Gave adequate information about the treatment and the expected progress.			
7. Gave the client an opportunity to participate in setting treatment goals.			
8. Insured the treatment was designed to meet client needs.			
9. Gave a between-session assignment to the client that matched the clients needs.			

REFERENCES

Clark CC. (1996). *Wellness Practitioner, Concepts, Research, and Strategies.* New York: Springer Publishing Company.

Collinge W. (1996). *The American Holistic Health Association Complete Guide to Alternative Medicine*. New York: Warner Books.

Krieger D. (1994). Advanced Therapeutic Touch Workshop. St. Petersburg, FL: Annual Convention, Nurse Healers Professional Associates, Don CeSar Hotel.

McKay M, Davis M, & Fanning P. (1995). *Messages, the Communication Book*. 2nd ed. Oakland, CA: New Harbinger.

5

GUIDELINES FOR CHOOSING THE RIGHT THERAPY

To be successful when integrating complementary therapies into practice, it is important to consider treatment goals, client and practitioner preferences and comfort levels, and practitioner expertise in a particular therapy.

When deciding which complementary practice to use, consider the following:

1.   Learn as much as possible about a particular complementary procedure before integrating it into practice. Besides taking a course in the subject, review current research findings. Unless referring the client to a complementary therapist, try out the procedure with nonclients. Find colleagues, family, or friends on whom you can hone your skills. Practice asking your simulated clients what they know about the procedure and then correcting misconceptions. Be sure to do this gently. Tell your simulated clients what the procedure entails, your experience using it, which conditions it has been effective with, how it might fit into their treatment plan, and any possible side effects or adverse reactions. Answer any questions they may have. Be sure to answer each one honestly and directly, remembering that as clients they will be anxious about any new procedure. Remind them that comfort level and enhanced results frequently increase as treatment progresses. Ask your simulated clients for feedback on your expertise, including what you said to them, how you said it, how you performed the procedure, and what other behaviors they would suggest that might improve your technique. (Use the information in Table 4.5, Chapter 4 to evaluate your simulated treatment session.)

2.   Determine your goals for using the therapy. What advantages does the procedure have for this client? Is the procedure being used primarily to maintain health, deal with chronic symptoms, reduce acute symptoms, or for some other reason?

3. Ask yourself which of the various complementary procedures best suits your goals and your client's goals. Build confidence by checking with more experienced colleagues.

4. Identify your comfort level. Ask yourself how comfortable you are with each possible procedure. Ask your clients how comfortable they are with trying each complementary procedure you are considering. Find out if clients have tried the procedure before and what their experience was with it.

Table 5.1 identifies appropriate complementary care approaches for each condition that have been identified by expert complementary practitioners. Use it as a reference source when beginning to integrate complementary procedures into practice. More detail on each recommended therapy can be found in later chapters in this book and other sources. In time, begin to combine therapies for a more powerful effect. For example, therapeutic touch often results in faster results for clients when it is combined with guided imagery.

Table 5.1   Choosing the Right Complementary Therapy

Condition	Suggested Complementary Procedures
AIDS	Affirmations, Chinese healing, coping skills training, exercise, guided imagery, herbs, hypnosis, nutrition/supplements, refuting irrational ideas, relaxation, thought stopping, touch therapies
Allergies	Affirmations, Ayurveda, Chinese healing, coping skills training, Feng Shui, guided imagery, herbs, hypnosis, lifestyle changes, nutrition/supplements, sound/music, touch therapies
Alzheimer's	Herbs, lifestyle changes, nutrition/supplements, sound/music
Anger/Aggression	Affirmations, aromatherapy, art/ritual, assertiveness, breathing, coping skills, exercise, hypnosis, journal writing, lifestyle changes, nutrition/supplements, refuting irrational ideas, sound/music
Anxiety/Panic	Affirmations, aromatherapy, art/ritual, Ayurveda, breathing, coping skills, exercise, hypnosis, journal writing, lifestyle changes, nutrition/supplements, refuting irrational ideas, relaxation therapy, sound/music, thought stopping, touch therapies
Appetite disturbance	Affirmations, aromatherapy, Feng Shui, nutrition/supplements, touch therapies
Arthritis	Affirmations, aromatherapy, assertiveness, Ayurveda, Chinese healing, exercise, lifestyle changes, nutrition/supplements, sound/music, touch therapies
Asthma	Affirmations, aromatherapy, breathing, Chinese healing, exercise, guided imagery, lifestyle change, music, nutrition/supplements, relaxation therapy, touch therapies

(continued)

Table 5.1   *(continued)*

Condition	Suggested Complementary Procedures
Attention Deficit Disorder	Affirmations, aromatherapy, breathing, Feng Shui, exercise, guided imagery, herbs, lifestyle change, nutrition/supplements, sound/music, touch therapies
Back pain	Affirmations, Ayurveda, aromatherapy, Chinese healing, coping skill, exercise, guided imagery, herbs, hypnosis, lifestyle changes, meditation, nutrition/supplements, sound/music, touch therapies
Balance/Falls	Affirmations, coping skills, exercise, guided imagery, herbs, lifestyle changes, nutrition/supplements, touch therapies
Bladder Infections	Affirmations, aromatherapy, herbs, lifestyle changes, nutrition/supplements, sound/music, touch therapies
Breast pain	Affirmations, herbs, lifestyle changes, nutrition/supplements, touch therapies
Bronchitis	Affirmations, aromatherapy, Ayurveda, guided imagery, herbs, lifestyle changes, nutrition/supplements, touch therapies
Burns	Aromatherapy, herbs, nutrition/supplements, sound/music
Bursitis	Affirmations, aromatherapy, herbs
Cancer	Affirmations, aromatherapy, art/ritual, assertiveness, Ayurveda, exercise, guided imagery, hypnotherapy, herbs, lifestyle changes, nutrition/supplements, relaxation therapy, sound/music, touch therapies
Candidiasis	Affirmations, aromatherapy, Ayurveda, herbs, lifestyle change, nutrition/supplements
Carpal Tunnel Syndrome	Exercise, herbs, lifestyle changes, nutrition/supplements, touch therapies
Cataract	Affirmations, nutrition/supplements
Cerebral Palsy	Sound/music
Chest pain	Ayurveda, breathing, guided imagery, hypnosis, nutrition/supplements, touch therapies
Cholesterol	Affirmations, Ayurveda, exercise, herbs, lifestyle changes, nutrition/supplements
Chronic Fatigue	Affirmations, aromatherapy, breathing, Chinese healing, exercise, herbs, lifestyle changes, nutrition/supplements, refuting irrational ideas, sound/music, touch therapies
Colds/Viruses	Affirmations, aromatherapy, assertiveness, guided imagery, herbs, lifestyle changes, nutrition/supplements, sound/music, touch therapies
Constipation	Ayurveda, aromatherapy, assertiveness, exercise, guided imagery, nutrition/supplements, sound/music, touch therapies

Table 5.1 *(continued)*

Condition	Suggested Complementary Procedures
Cough	Affirmations, aromatherapy, assertiveness, herbs, nutrition/supplements, refuting irrational ideas, touch therapies
Depression	Affirmations, aromatherapy, assertiveness, art/ritual, Ayurveda, breathing, exercise, guided imagery, herbs, hypnosis, lifestyle changes, meditation, nutrition/supplements, refuting irrational ideas, relaxation therapy, sound/music, touch therapies
Dermatitis	Affirmations, aromatherapy, assertiveness, Chinese healing, guided imagery, hypnosis, lifestyle changes, nutrition/supplements
Diabetes	Affirmations, Ayurveda, exercise, guided imagery, herbs, hypnosis, meditation, nutrition/supplements, sound/music, touch therapies
Diarrhea	Affirmations, aromatherapy, Ayurveda, exercise, herbs, nutrition/supplements, sound/music, touch therapies
Digestion	Affirmations, aromatherapy, Ayurveda, breathing, guided imagery, herbs, hypnosis, touch therapies
Diverticulosis	Affirmations, guided imagery, nutrition/supplements, touch therapies
Earache	Affirmations, aromatherapy, Ayurveda, exercises, herbs, lifestyle changes, nutrition/supplements
Eczema	Affirmations, aromatherapy, Ayurveda, Chinese healing, herbs, hypnosis, nutrition/supplements
Edema	Affirmations, exercise, nutrition/supplements, touch therapies
Endometriosis	Affirmations, exercise, herbs, lifestyle changes, nutrition/supplements, touch therapies
Esophagitis	Affirmations, guided imagery, herbs, hypnosis
Fatigue	Affirmations, herbs, touch therapies
Fever	Affirmations, Ayurveda, herbs, lifestyle changes, nutrition/supplements, touch therapies
Flatulence	Ayurveda, exercise, guided imagery, herbs, nutrition/supplements, touch therapies
Gallstones	Affirmations, Ayurveda, guided imagery, nutrition/supplements
Glaucoma	Affirmations, exercise, herbs, nutrition/supplements, touch therapies
Gout	Affirmations, herbs, lifestyle changes, nutrition/supplements, touch therapies
Grief	Affirmations, aromatherapy, breathing, exercise, coping skills, guided imagery, nutrition/supplements, sound/music, touch therapies

(continued)

Table 5.1 *(continued)*

Condition	Suggested Complementary Procedures
Gum Disease	Affirmations, aromatherapy, exercise, guided imagery, herbs, hypnosis, lifestyle changes, nutrition/supplements, touch therapies
Hay Fever	Affirmations, Ayurveda, exercise, guided imagery, nutrition/supplements, touch therapies
Headache	Affirmations, aromatherapy, assertiveness, Ayurveda, breathing, exercise, guided imagery, herbs, hypnosis, lifestyle factors, nutrition/supplements, sound/music, touch therapies
Heart Disease	Affirmations, aromatherapy, Ayurveda, breathing, Chinese healing, exercise, herbs, lifestyle changes, meditation, nutrition/supplements, relaxation therapy, sound/music, support group, touch therapies
Hemorrhoids	Affirmations, aromatherapy, assertiveness, exercise, guided imagery, herbs, nutrition/supplements, touch therapies
Herpes Virus	Affirmations, aromatherapy, lifestyle change, nutrition/supplements
Hypertension	Affirmations, aromatherapy, assertiveness, breathing, exercise, guided imagery, herbs, hypnosis, lifestyle changes, nutrition/supplements, sound/music, touch therapies
Immune disorders	Affirmations, Chinese healing, exercise, herbs, lifestyle changes, nutrition/supplements
Incontinence	Affirmations, exercise, nutrition/supplements
Indigestion	Affirmations, Ayurveda, aromatherapy, breathing, herbs, lifestyle changes, nutrition/supplements, touch therapies
Infection	Affirmations, aromatherapy, assertiveness, guided imagery, herbs, nutrition/supplements, touch therapies
Insect Bites	Aromatherapy, herbs, lifestyle changes, nutrition/supplements
Insomnia	Affirmations, aromatherapy, breathing, exercise, guided imagery, herbs, hypnosis, lifestyle changes, meditation, nutrition/supplements, sound/music
Irritable Bowel	Affirmations, exercise, guided imagery, herbs, relaxation therapy, hypnosis, nutrition/supplements, touch therapies
Kidney/Stones	Affirmations, aromatherapy, assertiveness, Chinese healing, exercise, guided imagery, lifestyle changes, nutrition/supplements, sound/music, touch therapies
Laryngitis	Affirmations, aromatherapy, assertiveness, Ayurveda, breathing, Chinese healing, herbs, lifestyle changes, nutrition/supplements
Liver imbalances	Affirmations, aromatherapy, assertiveness, Ayurveda, exercises, nutrition/supplements

Table 5.1 *(continued)*

Condition	Suggested Complementary Procedures
Memory	Affirmations, aromatherapy, breathing, guided imagery, herbs, hypnotherapy, nutrition/supplements, touch therapies
Meniere's Disease	Affirmation, aromatherapy, exercise, nutrition/supplements, touch therapies
Menopause	Affirmations, aromatherapy, exercise, guided imagery, herbs, lifestyle changes, meditation, nutrition/supplements, sound/music
Multiple Sclerosis	Affirmations, assertiveness, exercise, guided imagery, hypnosis, nutrition/supplements
Nausea	Aromatherapy, breathing, herbs, nutrition/supplements, touch therapies
Neuralgia	Affirmations, exercise, herbs, nutrition/supplements
Osteoporosis	Exercise, guided imagery, herbs, nutrition/supplements
Overweight	Affirmations, assertiveness, Ayurveda, breathing, exercise, guided imagery, nutrition/supplements
Pain	Affirmations, aromatherapy, assertiveness, breathing, exercise, guided imagery, herbs, hypnotherapy, lifestyle changes, meditation, music, nutrition/supplements, relaxation therapy, sound/music, touch therapies
Parkinson's Disease	Ayurveda, exercise, guided imagery, nutrition/supplements, sound/music
PMS	Affirmations, aromatherapy, exercise, guided imagery, herbs, lifestyle changes, nutrition/supplements, touch therapies
Pneumonia	Affirmations, aromatherapy, breathing, herbs, lifestyle changes, nutrition/supplements, touch therapies
Poisoning	Herbs, touch therapies
Pregnancy	Affirmations, exercise, herbs, nutrition/supplements, touch therapies
Prostate	Affirmations, assertiveness, Chinese healing, exercise, guided imagery, herbs, nutrition/supplements
Respiratory disorders	Affirmations, aromatherapy, breathing, Chinese healing, guided imagery, herbs, hypnosis, meditation, nutrition/supplements, relaxation, sound/music, touch therapies
Sexual desire	Affirmations, aromatherapy, herbs, nutrition/supplements
Shingles	Affirmations, Ayurveda, Chinese healing, herbs, lifestyle changes, nutrition/supplements
Sinus congestion	Affirmations, aromatherapy, assertiveness, breathing, Ayurveda, guided imagery, herbs, lifestyle changes, nutrition/supplements, touch therapies

(continued)

Table 5.1 *(continued)*

Condition	Suggested Complementary Procedures
Skin disorders	Affirmations, aromatherapy, Chinese healing, guided imagery, herbs, hypnosis, meditation, nutrition/supplements, relaxation therapy, touch therapies
Sore throat	Affirmations, aromatherapy, assertiveness, breathing, herbs, lifestyle changes, nutrition/supplements, touch therapies
Stroke	Affirmations, sound/music
Substance abuse	Affirmations, exercise, guided imagery, herbs, hypnosis, meditation, nutrition/supplements, relaxation therapy, thought stopping
Surgery	Affirmations, assertiveness, guided imagery, hypnosis, nutrition/supplements, relaxation therapy, touch therapies
TMJ	Breathing, guided imagery, herbs, hypnotherapy, nutrition/supplements, relaxation therapy, touch therapies
Tonsilitis	Affirmations, assertiveness, aromatherapy, Ayurveda, Chinese healing, herbs, lifestyle changes
Toothache	Affirmations, aromatherapy, Ayurveda, Chinese healing, herbs, lifestyle changes, touch therapies
Trauma	Breathing, coping skills, guided imagery, herbs, nutrition/supplements, relaxation, sound/music, touch therapies
Ulcerative Colitis	Ayurveda, guided imagery, hypnosis, nutrition/supplements, relaxation therapy, touch therapies
Vaginal disorders	Affirmations, herbs, lifestyle changes, nutrition/supplements
Varicose veins	Affirmations, aromatherapy, exercise, guided imagery, herbs, nutrition/supplements, touch therapies
Warts	Affirmations, Chinese healing, guided imagery, herbs, nutrition/supplements
Weight Maintenance/ Loss	Affirmations, aromatherapy, breathing, exercise, guided imagery, herbs, nutrition/supplements
Wounds	Aromatherapy, guided imagery, nutrition/supplements, touch therapies

REFERENCES

Chiazzari S. (1998). *Colour Scents*. Essex: C.W. Daniel Company, Ltd.

Clark CC. (1996). *Wellness Practitioner, Concepts, Research, and Strategies*. New York: Springer Publishing Company.

Credit LP, Hartunian SG, & Nowak MJ. (1998). *Your Guide to Complementary Medicine*. Garden City Park, NY: Avery Publishing Group.

Mowrey DB. (1993). *Herbal Tonic Therapies*. New Canaan, CT: Keats Publishing.

Snyder M, & Lindquist R. (1998). *Complementary/Alternative Therapies in Nursing*. 3rd Edition. New York: Springer Publishing Company.

6

EVALUATING RESULTS

Complementary therapy effects can be evaluated in several ways. Practitioners are most concerned with the effect of a specific procedure on a specific client. Indicants of treatment success and practitioner and client evaluation methods are presented in this chapter.

INDICANTS OF TREATMENT SUCCESS

The results of some complementary treatments are immediately apparent. For example, there may be changes in mood, pain, or physiological state after breathing exercises, relaxation therapy, guided imagery, touch therapies, meditation, or hypnosis have been implemented. Nutrition, supplements, herbs, rituals, Feng Shui, journal writing, and lifestyle changes may take days or weeks or longer to demonstrate an effect.

One criterion for a successful guided imagery session is that the client feels hopeful, powerful, and optimistic after completing it (Collinge, 1996). In touch therapies, the practitioner can often see a change in the client's musculature and breathing, and a relaxation and flushing of the face as circulation improves (Krieger, 1993) and the general relaxation response takes over.

When using affirmations, thought stopping, or refutation of irrational ideas, the practitioner will begin to notice the client using fewer self-deprecating remarks and more positive self-affirming statements. Clients may bring art or journal productions to a session and tell the practitioner about any breakthroughs in health status they notice, or ask for further assistance with the method.

JOINT PRACTITIONER-CLIENT EVALUATION

Traditional methods of evaluating treatment results include practitioner's diagnosis, client's subjective report of symptoms, and laboratory tests/results. Because client input is valued in a complementary approach, an evaluation procedure using client responses is used. The practitioner inquires about client symptoms, and asks the client to rate each symptom prior to and after treatment. Table 6.1 provides a format for assessment, treatment, and evaluation for one client.

Current medications, supplements, nutrition, exercise, and sources of support are identified in the initial session. Additions or changes are identified and added to future treatment sheets. The practitioner asks the clients to rate each symptom from 1 (minimal effect) to 10 (unbearable) and writes the rating on the Assessment/Treatment/Evaluation sheet. Treatments used, and specific measures and intra-session client homework agreed on during the session are also recorded.

At the beginning of the next session, the practitioner checks with the client to insure homework was completed, ascertains any difficulties in completing the assignment, and suggests ways of overcoming roadblocks prior to the following session.

CLIENT EVALUATION

Because client input is so important in complementary treatment, documents for eliciting clients' evaluation is a priority. A few forms used to assist clients to self-evaluate their progress are presented. More are presented in Part II when individual therapies are discussed. Table 6.2 provides a Wellness Daily Diary that can be used to obtain client information over a period of days. Data has been filled in for a client diagnosed with fibromyalgia whose goal was to increase energy and lose weight.

In a complementary approach, thoughts and feelings are believed to affect physical states and vice versa. For that reason, a Thought/Feelings Diary can be an important part of a complementary practitioner's approach. Table 6.3 provides a format for client evaluation of thoughts and feelings and methods to change them. Data for a client with anger control difficulties is presented.

Table 6.1   Assessment/Treatment/Evaluation

Date: 8/24/99   Client: Jason Stimtrex   Session #: 5

Current Medications: *"The doctor is giving me IV antibiotics 6x/week for my sinus infection and asthma. He cut back my medications. Now I only get a sleeping pill, my blood pressure medicine and Xanax.*

Current Supplements: *garlic capsules 3x/day, vitamin E 400 IU/day, vitamin C 500 mg 3x/day, calcium/magnesium (1,500:750 mg) a day.*

Current Eating Plan: *Vegetarian: no wheat or white rice. Chicken or fish 3x week. "I like rice pudding—my wife makes it for me."*

Current Exercise Plan: *Walk daily x 40 minutes, yoga class 1x week.*

Current Sources of Support: *Wife and grown daughter, men's church group.*

Table 6.1   *(continued)*

Other: *dogs, Charlie & Izzie*

Goal: *"Get rid of sinus infection and diarrhea."*

RATING: MINIMAL . . . . UNBEARABLE

SYMPTOM 1: Sinus "headache"

Rating at beginning of session:	1	2	3	4	5	6	7	8	9	⑩
Rating at end of session:	1	2	③	4	5	6	7	8	9	10

SYMPTOM 2: "Cold feet" (diabetes)

Rating at beginning of session:	1	2	3	4	5	6	7	8	⑨	10
Rating at end of session:	1	2	3	④	5	6	7	8	9	10

SYMPTOM 3: "Upset stomach and diarrhea"

Rating at beginning of session:	1	2	3	4	5	6	7	8	9	⑩
Rating at end of session:	1	2	3	4	5	6	⑦	8	9	10

SYMPTOM 4: "Sore neck and shoulders"

Rating at beginning of session:	1	2	3	4	5	6	7	8	9	⑩
Rating at end of session:	①	2	3	4	5	6	7	8	9	10

SYMPTOM 5: "Floaters and sore eyes"

Rating at beginning of session:	1	2	3	4	5	6	7	⑧	9	10
Rating at end of session:	1	2	3	④	5	6	7	8	9	10

TREATMENTS:

affirmations: *I refuse to let anyone irritate me and breathe in peace and joy.*
   It's getting easier and easier to follow a healthy meal plan.
   I enjoy the taste of my food and digest it well.
aromatherapy: *peppermint oil to sinus area*
art/ritual:
assertiveness: *discussed trying role playing client-physician interactions during next session*
breathing: *practiced diaphragmatic breathing in session*
coping skills: *I will not allow this situation to upset me.*
exercise: *Encouraged client to continue exercise program.*
Feng Shui: *consider having the dogs sleep on the other side of the house from your bedroom*

(continued)

Table 6.1   *(continued)*

guided imagery: *Asked client to breathe in healing relaxing energy as a color; breathe out whatever it's time to let go of as another color; picturing a cool color or liquid soothing his "hot" face and neck.*

herbs:

hypnosis/suggestions:

meditation:

nutritional counseling: *suggested using soy milk and cheese as an alternative to dairy products that produce mucus; avoid cold beverages with meals*

relaxation therapy/tape:

refuting irrational ideas:

sound/music therapy: *played a relaxing audiotape of client's choice during session*

touch therapies: *Jin Shin jyutsu for sinus, stomach, large intestine, muscle tension; massage to face, neck and shoulders; therapeutic touch—full body treatment*

HOMEWORK:

affirmations: *gave client health meal plan affirmation on a 3 × 5 card and asked him to read it 20x/day*

art/ritual: *Draw your pain in your journal.*

breathing: *Continue practicing diaphragmatic breathing daily.*

coping skills:

exercise: *Continue exercise program.*

Feng Shui:

guided imagery: *asked client to picture a protective shield around him when he was in a stressful situation*

herbs: *read about milk thistle, probiotics, fenugreek, thyme and peppermint (gave client handouts) will discuss implementing them next session*

hypnosis/suggestions:

journal writing: *asked client to purchase a journal that appeals to him and begin writing about his feelings in family interactions*

meditation:

nutrition/supplementation:

relaxation therapy/tape:

refuting irrational ideas:

sound/music therapy:

touch therapies: *asked client to rub his wife's feet and ask her to massage his*

other:

additional notes:

Table 6.2 Wellness Daily Diary

Start Date: *Wednesday*
Stop Date: *Tuesday*

Date	Time	Food/Liquids/ Condiments	Bowel Movements (consistency, gas, bloating)	Activities (with whom for how long)	Symptoms and mood (include changes for 1 hour after eating and at any other time)	Vitamins/ Medications (include dosage once, then any changes)
Wed	*7:30 a.m.*	*orange juice* *coffee*	*gas* *bloating*	*arguing with son*		*multi-vitamin* *vitamin E 400 M*
	8:30 a.m.				*depressed*	
	9:30 a.m.			*boss gave me a terrible assignment*	*angry*	*2 Tylenol*
	10 a.m. *noon*	*Snickers* *burger & fries* *Coke*		*working on new project alone*	*pain all over* *tired, dizzy*	
	1 p.m.		*hard bowel movement*			
	3 p.m.	*2 mints*				
	3:30 p.m.				*tired*	
	3:45 p.m.	*coffee*				
	6:30 p.m.	*broiled chicken* *mashed potatoes and* *gravy* *apple*		*husband came home late*	*annoyed*	
	7 p.m.		*gas, indigestion*		*exhausted*	*Mylanta*

Table 6.3 Feelings Diary

Name: Date:

Date	Time	Setting	Conversations/ Thoughts	Feelings	Approaches Tried to Change Feelings	Results
10/12	9 a.m.	Work	Boss told me I wasn't producing. I think he's a dope.	rage	deep breathing guided imagery	At least I didn't punch him.
10/12	noon	cafeteria	Waitress told me there wasn't any fish. She's too lazy to get it.	real angry	Told myself it was irrational to think there was fish when maybe there wasn't.	I didn't cool down for an hour and that spoiled my lunch hour.
10/12	5 p.m.	Someone cut me off and I rolled down the window and told him what I thought.	rage	picturing him in his underwear	I laughed and realized what a jerk I was being.	

REFERENCES

Collinge W. (1996). *The American Holistic Health Association Complete Guide to Alternative Medicine.* New York: Warner Books.

Kreiger D. (1993). *Accepting Your Power to Heal, The Personal Practice of Therapeutic Touch.* Sante Fe, NM: Bear & Company.

7

STRENGTHS, COSTS AND INSURANCE COVERAGE

A major rationale for using complementary approaches is that they have strengths allopathic procedures do not. Another attractive feature of complementary procedures is that they are cost-effective. However, insurance coverage is not always available and clients may have to pay for some treatments out-of-pocket. This situation is changing rapidly, with HMOs adding new riders and coverages daily. This chapter explores the strengths, costs and insurance coverage for some complementary procedures.

STRENGTHS OF COMPLEMENTARY PROCEDURES

Chinese healing methods do well with colds, flu, headache, allergy and many chronic conditions that can bewilder allopathic practitioners. Clients often go to Chinese healers when they know something is wrong with them but are told by an allopathic practitioner: "We can't find anything wrong with you. Your lab tests are all normal. Maybe you need to see a psychiatrist."

It may be that the Chinese diagnostic methods are able to detect more subtle indicators of health and illness than allopathic methods. Chinese methods work at a preventive level, identifying a disorder prior to its manifestation in physical tissue (Collinge, 1996).

Some conditions such as chronic fatigue syndrome, fibromyalgia, food sensitivities, and environmental illnesses are poorly understood by allopathic practitioners. In the Chinese frame of reference, everything experienced by the client is believed to be meaningful and is fit into an overriding diagnostic view (Collinge, 1996).

Chinese healing methods are also used to supplement allopathic procedures. They can help speed recovery from surgery or deal with the side effects of chemotherapy or radiation treatment.

Like Chinese healing methods, Ayurveda is also focused on prevention. Its main aim is to prescribe regimens to maintain health and wellness, help clients attain higher levels of health, support the body's capacity for self-repair and extend the life span (Collinge, 1996).

The greatest contributions of mind-body approaches (breathing therapy, guided imagery, hypnosis, lifestyle change, meditation, and relaxation therapy) are in reducing stress-related and chronic conditions and in bringing relief for symptoms of acute illnesses and from treatments such as radiation, chemotherapy or surgery (Collinge, 1996).

Touch therapies work on any condition that benefits from greater blood circulation and the release of tension. Psychological conditions may also benefit due to physiological changes that help harmonize and rebalance hormonal and nervous systems (Collinge, 1996).

COMPLEMENTARY TREATMENT COSTS

Complementary procedures tend to be less expensive than allopathic treatment because they do not involve expensive modern laboratory testing, high-technology equipment, pharmaceuticals, or high malpractice insurance costs. Although some complementary practitioners may use or recommend nutritional supplements, herbal remedies, or essential oils, client fees are primarily for treatment time in the practitioner's office (Collinge, 1996).

Treatments in Ayurvedic and Chinese systems typically run from $50 to $100 for complementary practitioners, with charges higher for allopathic physicians. Herbs may add another $10 to $50 per month, depending on client symptoms. Appointments may be scheduled once or twice a week for several weeks. Procedures are characteristically spaced farther apart as time progresses, except for complex chronic conditions, which may require treatments over several months (Collinge, 1996).

Mind-body approaches, including hypnosis, relaxation therapy, and guided imagery, are even less expensive, because no herbs or other products are used. Fees for touch therapies tend to range from $30 to $80 an hour, with higher costs in urban areas and for specialty areas (Collinge, 1996).

INSURANCE COVERAGE

The findings from a survey of 156 HMOs by Landmark Health, Inc. were reported in 1996 (Chow). Landmark Health is a managed care company that offers complementary health care for its more than 3 million members nationwide. Seventy percent of the HMOs who responded to the survey reported an increase in requests for complementary therapies from their members. Fifty-eight percent of the responding HMOs indicated they planned to offer complementary therapies to their members in the next 2 years.

Other insurance companies are also beginning to cover complementary procedures. Some of the earliest to provide coverage were Oxford Health Plans (New

York, New Jersey, Connecticut, New Hampshire, and Pennsylvania), Alternative
Health Insurance Services (All states except California), Alternative Health Plan
(nationwide), Group Health Insurance Services (Western Washington), Mutual
of Omaha (Ornish lifestyle heart disease reversal program), Common Well Health
Plan (Eastern Massachusetts), Kaiser Foundation Health Plan (Northern California), American Western Life Insurance Wellness Plan (California, Oregon, Colorado, Utah, New Mexico, and Arizona), and Bienestar Gold (New York, New
Jersey, Connecticut, and Florida). Bienstar, among others, is rapidly expanding
into other parts of the country (Clark, 1996, 1997).

Other providers and insurers are adding complementary procedures to their
available services. Denver's largest managed care organization, Sloans Lake
Managed Care has added a complementary rider to its PPO and HMO plans
covering herbs, some touch therapies, Chinese healing, Ayurveda, and some
other therapies.

Axis HealthCare in Portland, Oregon has added naturopaths, acupuncturists,
and massage therapists to its panel of providers. Health Partners in Minnesota now
covers nutritional counseling, herbs, and some touch therapies (Villaire, 1998).

State reimbursement procedures are also changing. For example, in 1996, the
state of Washington passed a law requiring insurers to pay for visits for all
categories of health care providers licensed and certified by the state. This means
that complementary providers, if licensed or certified by the state, must be paid
by insurers (Wolfe, 1999).

Insurers are beginning to cover massage therapy. In cases where it is not
covered, licensure of the practitioner and an allopathic physician's prescription
may help (Collinge, 1996).

REFERENCES

Chow S. (1996). Health maintenance organizations and alternative medicine: A closer
look. Unpublished document by Landmark Healthcare.
Clark CC. (1996). From internet to insurance—alternative/complementary therapies on
the rise. Editorial. *Alternative Health Practitioner: The Journal of Complementary
and Natural Care* 2(3):155–156.
Clark CC. (1997). Wellness program offers direct access to complementary therapies.
Alternative Health Practitioner: The Journal of Complementary and Natural Care
3(3):155–156.
Collinge W. (1996). *The American Holistic Health Association Complete Guide to Alterna-
tive Medicine*. New York: Warner Books.
Villaire M. (1998). More health plans add alternative medicine coverage. *Alternative
Therapies* 4(3):27.
Wolfe K. (In press). Integrating complementary medicine into managed care. *Alternative
Health Practitioner: The Journal of Complementary and Natural Care*.

8

MARKETING A COMPLEMENTARY PRACTICE

This chapter explores basic marketing decisions and describes basic ways to attract clients to a complementary practice. Also included are suggestions for carving out a complementary practice market.

BASIC MARKETING AND BUSINESS DECISIONS

A marketing strategy is one part of a business plan, and a mission statement is the beginning of the process. Table 8.1 provides components for developing a mission statement. Check off the components after they have been completed.

Developing a primary marketing strategy provides focus for integration. Recommended methods include: specializing in one complementary procedure; becoming known as an expert complementary practitioner; using the Internet to

Table 8.1   Developing a Mission Statement for Integration

Component	Date Completed
Stated purpose of practice	_____
Primary elements of current practice	_____
Fit of complementary procedures with current practice	_____
Goals for integrating complementary procedures into current practice	_____
Overriding strategy for practice	_____
Unique characteristics of practice	_____
How uniqueness will be enhanced by adding complementary procedures	_____

advertise; offering wide range of services at a low fee; and forming a coalition with other complementary practitioners (Heller, 1997).

Integrating complementary procedures into a practice calls for a 3–5 year projection of what the practice should look like, identifying any expected changes that may be required to achieve the vision. Table 8.2 provides actions to take to assist integrating complementary procedures into practice. Check them off as they are completed.

Depending on the complementary procedures to be integrated, the following equipment will need to be purchased: blank tapes for making relaxation and guided imagery messages, dietary supplements, herbs, and new business cards and/or letterhead. Space will need to be located for display of new products and related client and practitioner reading material.

Belief in and knowledge of a practitioner's framework is a crucial factor in successful treatment outcomes (Heller, 1997). If the practitioner has published any articles or books on complementary topics, these can be displayed in the waiting room to reaffirm the decisions clients made to become part of the practice.

As complementary practice grows in importance, competition will increase. Practitioners must evaluate the strengths and limitations of their practice, evaluate the competition and the needs of the marketplace. The yellow pages and related directories of practitioners are a place to begin. Table 8.3 provides information for evaluating competing complementary practitioners.

The best course may be to network with other complementary practitioners, taking them to lunch and sharing information. Joining complementary practitioner groups may also provide valuable marketing information.

Table 8.2   Actions to Take to Integrate Complementary Procedures

Action	Date Completed
Set measurable goals for integrating complementary procedures into practice	_____
Choose tactics to achieve the goals	_____
Identify dates for achieving goals	_____
Make changes in emergency coverage	_____
Educate clerical staff regarding new procedures and forms	_____
Enhance accessibility of treatment setting	_____
Buy/arrange new furnishings	_____
Buy/arrange new equipment	_____
Develop new client handouts	_____
Develop new client payment procedures	_____
Develop new informed-consent forms	_____
Develop/revise release-of-information forms	_____
Change billing procedures	_____
Devise new treatment-record forms	_____

Table 8.3   Evaluating Competing Complementary Practices

Evaluation Area	Date Evaluated
Practitioners offering complementary services	_____
Types of services being offered	_____
Fees of other complementary practitioners	_____
Contracts of other complementary practitioners	_____
Complementary practitioner group meetings	_____

The passage of "any willing provider" in some states can affect marketing approaches. This legislation could increase the probability of obtaining clients for some complementary practitioners and reduce it for others. Knowledge gained from keeping informed of national and local changes will help shape marketing efforts.

Population trends, locally and nationally, should also be considered. Table 8.4 provides information for addressing these marketing issues. For each demographic aspect, develop a marketing strategy.

ATTRACTING CLIENTS

There are seven basic ways to attract new clients to a complementary practice: advertising, provider referrals, central or organization referrals, conventions/ annual meetings of related organizations, health food store networking, provider-based seminars, and word-of-mouth referrals.

Advertising

Advertising in publications read by clients interested in complementary practices is an important marketing procedure. As bias against health care provider advertis-

Table 8.4   Demographic Considerations

Demographic Aspect	Marketing Strategy
Traditional families	_____
Nontraditional families	_____
Adolescent population	_____
Children	_____
Older adults	_____
Cultural diversity	_____
Symptoms/conditions	_____
Commercial/residential mix	_____

ing decreases, mass media will probably become an important vehicle for complementary practice marketing (Gordon & Silverstein, 1998).

Cable television, health-related radio and local talk shows provide venues for marketing complementary practitioner services. The curriculum vitae is a holdover from academia, but a business resume is more likely to be understood and used by the media. The first page should emphasize unique characteristics or accomplishments of the practitioner, preferably related to job history. Educational history appears at the end of the resume. Any media experiences belong near the front if the resume is being sent to the media as a public relations tool.

Another media-related marketing tool is the newsletter. Practitioner-generated newsletters can provide information about a complementary practice while educating noncomplementary practitioners and potential clients about the use and effectiveness of a particular procedure. The Internet is a relatively new marketing tool that deserves consideration and investigation.

One of the oldest and most useful methods of attracting clients is the use of a business card, letterhead, and brochure. A logo conveys an image of the practice, while a tag line can point out something unique about a practice, for example: "Using relaxation therapy to prepare adults for surgery," or "Guided Imagery Specialists," or "Your community specialist in nutrition and dietary supplements."

Although not strictly advertising, sending out press releases about integrating complementary procedures into a practice may bring a call from a local newspaper for an interview. Referrals and other interviews could follow. Copies of published articles, a business resume or biographical summary, and clippings of other relevant newspaper articles written about the practitioner should be sent as part of the news release packet. The address and phone number of the practitioner must be included.

Friends, colleagues, and family members need to be alerted about a practitioner's decision to integrate complementary procedures into a practice. Referrals could result.

Provider Referrals

Complementary practitioners need to devise ways to develop referral relationships with allopathic providers. One study (Borkan, Neher, Anson, & Smoker, 1994) revealed that 55% to 77% of the allopathic practitioners surveyed referred clients to complementary providers. In order of frequency, their reasons for referring were: patient request, patient cultural beliefs, lack of patient response to allopathic treatment, and belief the patient had a "nonorganic" or "psychological" problem.

These reasons for referral could be the start of marketing to allopathic practitioners to enhance a complementary practitioner's practice base. Brochures, business cards, and personal meetings could be used to reinforce the reasons for referring a patient to a complementary practitioner.

Another likely referral possibility are the allopathic practitioners who practice holistic medicine. They are the most likely to refer to complementary practitioners because their belief structure and practice is most in tune with a complementary approach. Such relationships need to be cultivated.

Central or Organization Referrals

Complementary and allopathic practitioners can investigate central or organizational referral sources. Managed care plans and insurers in surrounding geographical areas may have established formalized referral relationships with complementary providers. Often, they publish directories for their customers. By becoming a local provider, chances of obtaining referrals can be increased.

Becoming active in community religious, health, civic, or business groups is rewarding and enhances the image of the provider as a giving and caring person. It also provides opportunities to meet people who may become potential referral sources.

Volunteering to teach a class on complementary therapies at a school, medical center, library, or support group meeting for a chronic illness can put the practitioner in the public eye.

Organizations such as the American Holistic Medical Association, the American Holistic Nurses Association, and the Nurse Healers Cooperative (among others) publish directories of their members. Complementary practitioners can join these organizations and enhance the likelihood of being contacted by practitioners in other states who are looking for referral sources for clients who are relocating. Schools providing education for complementary practitioners may also provide referrals (see Appendix for more information).

Participating in Conventions/Annual Meetings of Related Organizations

When contacting organizations to obtain their directories, complementary practitioners can inquire about conventions and annual conferences. By identifying meetings in the general vicinity of the practitioner's office and then offering to present a speech on a topic related to services offered, the word can be spread about a practice. By writing their own biographical summaries and asking the person introducing speakers to read it, complementary practitioners can insure important practice information will not be overlooked in the tension of the moment. If feasible, an ad can be placed in the convention's program. Purchased booth space in the display area can also provide an opportunity for demonstrating one or more services and handing out brochures and business cards. Depending on the practitioner's marketing beliefs, discount or free initial consultation cards can also be handed out.

Health Food Stores

An overwhelming percentage of people make their first visit to a health food store in the midst of a health crisis (Emerich, 1996). Their short-term purpose may be to buy supplements or herbs, but their long-term goal is to enhance wellness (Anderson, 1996).

Health food stores often offer programs related to complementary practices to their customers. Many look for speakers with expertise in related areas and have bulletin boards and lists of complementary practitioners they make available to their clientele. Making friends with health food store owners and managers may be a good marketing tool for complementary practitioners.

Provider-Based Seminars

In addition to speaking at conventions and health food stores, complementary practitioners can develop their own seminars for potential clientele. Seminars can be offered for free at the practitioner's office or advertised for a fee at a nearby holistic center or spa. Some newspapers will advertise upcoming seminars at no charge in their health supplements; others charge a fee.

Word-of-Mouth Referrals

Word-of-mouth is perhaps the best referral system. To enhance word-of-mouth referrals, quality of services must be examined (Heller, 1997). Table 8.5 provides information for evaluating quality of services.

Clients who come to practitioners through word-of-mouth referrals are usually more motivated and believe they can find help. They generally trust the referral person or organization and are more apt to trust the complementary practitioner who was referred. Once a complementary practitioner becomes established, this form of finding clientele increases in importance. Becoming well known in a community as a helpful and effective practitioner means referrals will most likely increase. By offering to be on boards of directors of holistic centers or related health care organizations, complementary practitioners enhance their chances of having clients referred to them by their board of colleagues.

CARVING OUT A COMPLEMENTARY PRACTICE MARKET

It will be easiest to carve out a complementary practice market if the following benefits are available (Colgate, 1995):

1. Services are presented as complementary to, not alternative for, allopathic treatments.
2. Protocols elucidate specific treatment procedures.
3. Cost comparisons to allopathic procedures are available for similar conditions.
4. Research is available to show that the complementary practice is effective.

Table 8.5 Evaluating Quality of Services

Considerations	Date Evaluation Completed
Time Considerations	
1. Is adequate time allowed for appointments?	_____
2. Is adequate time allowed between appointments to answer important phone calls?	_____
3. Is there adequate time between sessions to complete treatment notes?	_____
4. Is there sufficient time between sessions to allow for practitioner recovery and reflection?	_____
Investment in Continuing Education	
1. Is there time to read complementary journals and books?	_____
2. Is there time to attend relevant workshops and seminars?	_____
Quality Record Keeping	
1. Is there a plan in place for what happens to complementary client records if the practitioner dies or becomes incapacitated?	_____
2. Does record keeping include collecting client feedback?	_____
3. Is outcome data on complementary procedures available?	_____
4. Is there a follow-up survey in place, preferably administered at the end of treatment and 3 and/or 6 months afterward?	_____
5. Is there a record in place to summarize geographical, age, gender, symptoms, length of treatment, and referral sources to allow for analysis of practice?	_____

5. Malpractice insurance is carried.
6. The practitioner is licensed or certified in the procedures offered.

Some elements that reduce the effectiveness of complementary marketing are:

1. There is a lack of coordination of care with primary care providers.
2. Services are not well managed or identified.
3. Prospective clients are not aware of or interested in obtaining the complementary service.

Developing a Marketing Plan

A marketing plan states specific objectives for the coming year, and strategies for accomplishing those goals. Objectives envole from a mission statement and include a measure of evaluation, for example, to increase using complementary procedures by 10%, to increase revenues from complementary procedures by 20%, or to increase net after-tax profits by 15% (Heller, 1997).

Some common marketing goals are presented in Table 8.6. The information can be used to develop specific goals.

Table 8.6 Developing a One-Year Marketing Plan

Goals	Time allotted per week	Percentage increase expected
Increasing profits	_____	_____
Increasing referrals	_____	_____
Providing related workshops	_____	_____
Developing a new brochure	_____	_____
Networking with practitioners	_____	_____
Identifying sources of capital to accomplish integration	_____	_____
Collecting client outcome data	_____	_____
Giving free complementary lectures	_____	_____
Writing about complementary practices	_____	_____
Developing a complementary consultation service	_____	_____
Placing complementary practice ads in relevant publications	_____	_____

REFERENCES

Anderson M. (1996). Larry Dossey MD is finding common ground between alternative and conventional medicine. *Natural Foods Merchandiser* 17(3):48–52.

Borkan J, Neher JO, Anson O, & Smoker B. (1994). Referrals for alternative therapies. *Journal of Family Practice* 39:545–550.

Colgate MA. (1995). Gaining insurance coverage for alternative therapies. *Journal of Health Care Marketing* 15(1):24–28.

Emerich M. (1996). Industry growth: 22.6%. *Natural Foods Merchandiser* 17(6):1,22.

Gordon R, & Silverstein G. (1998). Marketing channels for alternative health care. In R Gordon, BC Nienstedt, and WM Gesler (Eds.), *Alternative Therapies* (pp. 87–103). New York: Springer Publishing Company.

Heller KM. (1997). *Strategic Marketing*. Sarasota, FL: Professional Resource Exchange.

PART II

HOW TO INTEGRATE SELECTED COMPLEMENTARY THERAPIES

A

Nutrition, Herbs, and Essential Oils

9

NUTRITION AND SUPPLEMENTS

A 1998 study of medical and nonmedical providers of asthma care found that both groups identified dietary and nutritional approaches as the most prevalent and useful asthma treatment option. The predominance of diet and nutrition supplementation used by MDs and non-MDs suggests that research and education should be directed toward this area of complementary practice (Davis, Gold, Hackman, Stern, & Gershwin, 1998).

As early as 1977, the Senate Select Committee on Nutrition and Human Needs associated poor nutrition with 6 of the 10 causes of death: heart disease, some cancers, stroke and hypertension, diabetes, arteriosclerosis, and cirrhosis of the liver.

GUIDELINES FOR READING NUTRITIONAL INFORMATION

Some guidelines to keep in mind when reading nutritional information include:

1. Determine the author's background, specificity, and comprehensiveness of references. All authors have biases; be sure you know which ones the author you are reading has. Many authors do not use complete references, up-to-date references, or only include references supporting their point of view; determine as much as possible which variables are operating.
2. Go back to the original reference whenever possible to determine unreliable reporting.
3. Determine the source of funding of the periodical or book; e.g., if food producers are funders, question whether the results or types of research being reported may be biased.
4. Read as many different kinds of nutritional information as possible in order to get a balanced view of the issues.
5. When a relatively nonbiased source is found, keep returning to it for information in the future and tell clients about it.

Tables 9.1 and 9.2 can help clients evaluate nutritional wellness.

FOOD MYTHS

Be aware of food myths that are held by clients. Some of the most frequently found are:

1. *Meat contains more protein than other foods.* Actually, meat contains only about 25% protein and is about in the middle of the protein quantity scale, ranking below soybeans, fish, milk, soybean flour, and eggs.

2. *Large quantities of meat must be eaten to provide sufficient protein to grow and replace body tissues.* Most Americans eat twice the amount of protein their bodies can use; the recommended daily allowance of protein, 50–60 grams, can be reached even when all meat, fish, and poultry are eliminated from the diet. The daily protein requirements of a 170-pound man doing light work is 25 to 30 grams. A bowl of pea or bean soup, a slice of whole grain bread, and a vegetable salad supplies all the protein he needs (Balch & Balch, 1990). For example, by combining wheat and beans, milk and rice, milk and peanuts, or beans and rice, dishes containing all the amino acids necessary for the body can be obtained. Additionally all soybean products such as tofu and tempeh are

Table 9.1   Signs of Balanced Eating

Check for signs of balanced eating by observing the presence of the following:

- good endurance and high energy level
- alertness and responsiveness with good attention span
- shiny, lustrous hair
- healthy scalp
- thyroid gland of normal size
- clear, bright eyes
- lack of circles or puffiness around eyes
- moist lips of good color
- pink tongue with papillae present
- pink, firm gums
- clean, straight teeth
- smooth, slightly moist skin
- flat abdomen
- well-developed legs and feet
- lack of tenderness, weakness, or swelling in legs or feet
- normal weight for height, age, and body build
- erect posture with straight back, arms, legs, abdomen in chest slightly out
- well-developed, firm muscles
- feelings of calm
- good appetite and digestion
- easy and regular elimination
- sleeping well

Table 9.2   What Does Your Body Need?

Because of conflicting opinions and views on nutrition, a useful approach is to ask clients to assume their bodies know what they need and will begin to show signs when they are not adequately nourished. Ask clients to begin to chart their reactions to various foods by asking the following questions:

1. How well does this food seem to go through my digestive system? Does this food seem to be soothing or cleansing or health-promoting?
2. How do I sleep after ingesting this food?
3. What sort of stool is produced the day after I eat this food?
4. How are my breath and body odor the day after I eat this food?
5. How is my energy level the day of and the day after I eat this food?
6. How does what I am eating affect my skin, hair, and fingernails?
7. How does what I am eating affect my body shape and weight?
8. How does what I am eating affect my ability to concentrate?
9. How does what I am eating affect my relationships with others?
10. How does what I am eating affect how I feel about me and my life?

---

complete proteins. Fortifying cornmeal with the amino acid, lysine, also results in a complete protein. Strict vegetarians must remember to supplement their intake with vitamin B_{12} which is found only in meat (Balch & Balch, 1990).

3. *Meat offers the highest quality protein available.* Quality of protein refers to amount of protein available that is usable by the body; eggs and milk are more usable by the body than meat is, and soybeans and whole rice are as usable (Lappe, 1975).

4. *Sugar is sugar.* Sugar occurs naturally in milk, fruits, and vegetables; although sugar is being eaten in the food, it is being ingested with fiber, minerals, vitamins, and proteins, thus providing a superior combination of nutrients as compared to processed sugars in candy, sodas, and other sweets.

5. *Sugar is a good source of energy.* Refined sugar leads to less energy because the food is digested quickly, and the blood level of sugar (glucose) rises very rapidly. As a result, insulin is released in excess into the blood, and liver reserves of glycogen (stored glucose) are used, leading to fatigue, shakiness, irritability, faintness, and (in some people) violent behavior. Eating refined sugar results in highs and lows, and more coffee (with sugar) or another soda or piece of candy are then used to get a "lift." For high energy, frequent, high-protein meals or complex carbohydrates such as grains or vegetables are recommended.

6. *Starchy foods put on weight.* Complex carbohydrates such as whole grain pasta, baked potatoes, unrefined rice, and whole grain breads and cereals contain a great deal of fiber that is filling; it is only when butter, margarine, sour cream, or other fillings or toppings are used that calories accrue.

Weight Maintenance

Basal metabolism decreases at a rate of 2% to 5% with every decade past the age of 30, so activity may be the only safe way to diminish the accumulation of fat that is normal with aging (Bennett & Gurin, 1982, p. 252). Studies of populations who are vigorously active also end credence to the argument that exercise lowers set point. For example, Norwegian woodcutters do not grow fat with age; they maintain about 15% body fat for 40 years (Skobak-Kaczynski & Andersen, 1975).

If the theory is correct, people should lose weight spontaneously when undertaking an exercise program without dieting. Gwinup worked with a group of obese men and women to test the theory. All participants had been discouraged by repeated failures at dieting. The researcher told the group to forget about what they ate and begin a program of physical activity. Most began with brisk walking for 10 or 15 minutes daily. Although most subjects dropped out, all who reached the point of walking briskly for at least 30 min. 5 days/week lost weight.

The 11 women who stayed with the program chose to increase their activity and within 1 1/2 years each lost 22 lb. on the average and continued a steady, slow loss. The benefits of losing weight in this manner are that there are no negative effects of dieting, including: weakness, increased nervousness, feelings of deprivation, loss of muscle, or quick release of fat-stored toxins into the bloodstream. More than a third of the weight lost during dieting and two thirds lost during a fast reflect loss of muscle, not fat (Gwinup, 1975).

Exercise alone is a slow route to weight loss; about one third of a pound is lost per week for the overweight or obese and one tenth of a pound per week for people with ideal weight (Epstein & Wing, 1980). Frequency of exercise is important in weight loss. People who exercise 4 or 5 times a week lose weight three times faster than those who exercise 3 days a week; exercising once or twice a week has *no* effect on weight loss (Epstein & Wing, 1980). So much for the weekend athlete syndrome.

A recent study comparing lean to obese men and women found that both groups consumed the same number of calories. What differed was the amount of fat, added sugar, and fiber. Obese people derived a greater part of their energy intake from fat, a greater percentage of their sugar intake from added sugar, and a lower intake of fiber than lean people (Miller et al., 1994). Alterations in diet composition rather than number of calories ingested may have been an important weight control strategy for overweight adults.

The type of food eaten, important to weight loss, is even more important to wellness. Combining an exercise program with a very low carbohydrate diet is not wise; carbohydrates are needed to replenish the body's store of glycogen. Short-term, low-carbohydrate diets are incompatible with strenuous exercise; listlessness, dehydration, and acetone-breath are correlates of this kind of regime (Phinney et al., 1980).

Diabetes and Weight Loss

Although the reason is not completely understood, lowering the body's stores of fat leads to an increased sensitivity to insulin. Therefore, diabetes clients need to reduce their weight. The traditional low carbohydrate diet has been called into question. As long as the overall intake of calories is low enough to produce weight loss and large amounts of refined sugar are excluded, complex carbohydrates, especially whole grain foods, are desirable foods for weight loss plans (Simpson et al., 1981).

In general, whether seeking to prevent a chronic illness (or its complications) or to maintain a lean body, research provides evidence that a primarily vegetarian meal plan is best. Making complex carbohydrates the centerpiece of every meal—loading up on whole grains, fresh fruits and vegetables, and legumes—and decreasing fats and added sugars is the road to nutritional wellness.

Common Manifestations of Food Allergies

The following symptoms are often associated with food allergies (Balch & Balch, 1997): acne, especially pimples around the mouth or on the chin; arthritis; asthma; chest and shoulder pains; colitis; depression; fatigue; food cravings; headaches; hemorrhoids; insomnia; intestinal problems; muscle disorders; obesity; sinus problems; ulcers; unexplained weight change; bedwetting; conjunctivitis; diarrhea; dizzy spells and floating sensations; excessive drooling; dark circles under the eyes; puffy eyes; fluid retention; eye pain or tearing; nasal congestion or chronic runny nose; noises in the ear; hyperactivity; hearing loss; phobias; blurred vision that comes and goes; poor memory or concentration; red circles on the cheeks; poor muscle coordination; sensitivity to light; swollen fingers and cold hands; unusual body odor; recurrence of illness despite treatment; severe menstrual symptoms; sensitivity to light; repeated colds or ear infections especially in children; acid/alkaline imbalance; and anemia.

Food allergies usually develop slowly. The body eventually forms an intolerance to foods consumed daily. Avoiding an allergenic food for 60 to 90 days usually clears the body of any toxic reaction. A rotation diet can be used at that point: consume a food no more frequently than once every 4 days. Before starting a rotation regime, Balch and Balch (1997) recommend a fresh fruit juice and fresh vegetable juice fast.

The best juices for a blood purification fast are lemon, beet, carrot, and all leafy green vegetables. The latter contain chlorophyll that cleanses the blood of impurities, but also builds up the blood with important nutrients and inhibits cellular damage from radiation (Balch & Balch, 1997).

For clients who exhibit any of the allergic symptoms, it may be useful to do either pulse or muscle testing. Directions follow for both.

Pulse Testing.   If clients suspect they are allergic to a specific food or supplement, they can be taught how to take their pulse before and 15 to 20 minutes after ingesting a substance. If the pulse rate increases more than 10 beats per minute, the food or supplement is omitted from the diet for 1 month, and then retested.

Muscle Testing.   Another way to test substances for their appropriateness is muscle testing. This test requires two people. The practitioner stands in front of and facing the client and uses the following directions to muscle test:

1. Ask the client to hold the right (or left) arm straight out at shoulder level and think "strong." Push down firmly on the client's extended wrist with the palm of your hand, then release. This is the baseline measure for strength.
2. Ask the client to hold the substance against the chest at the level of the thymus and think "strong," while holding the same arm as before extended at shoulder level.
3. Push down on the wrist again in the same spot. If the client cannot hold the arm at shoulder level, it is considered a "weak" test result and a negative substance for the client to ingest at that time.

NUTRITIONAL INTERVENTIONS

When using nutritional interventions with clients, use the following guidelines:

1. Start with a small dose of a food or supplement and then assess the results before building to a higher dose or continuing on.
2. Rashes, stomach upsets, opposite reactions to those intended are examples of symptoms clients should be asked to report.
3. Muscle testing or a pulse test can be used to double check if a substance tests positive for clients.

Client Handouts

Use the following information as handouts for clients.

Breakfast in the car, fast food for lunch, and a dinner meeting . . . a lifestyle of eating on the go. Here are some tips for healthy habits when you are away from home, from the National Center for Nutrition and Dietetics.

The Choice Is Yours

- The type of restaurant you select affects the amount of control you will have over food choices. A full service restaurant offers the most flexibility. Cafeterias allow you to control portion sizes and toppings like gravy, sauce, and salad dressing.
- Do not be afraid to ask questions about how a dish is prepared and whether lower fat substitutions are available.

Less Fat, Still Fast

- Fast food chains are jumping on the low fat bandwagon—look for low fat dairy products and hearty healthy grilled chicken or lean meat entrees.

Table 9.3 can help clients achieve their ideal weight.

Table 9.3   Getting to Your Ideal Weight

The idea that your mind controls your body is not new, but how many of us tap our considerable mind power to enhance our wellness? Positive affirmation and visualization can be combined to obtain your ideal weight. Before each meal, try the following exercise:

Step One: Find a quiet, peaceful spot and spend 5 minutes relaxing your body. Keep your eyes closed throughout the exercise.

Step Two: Say, "I see and feel my body as I want it to look and feel." Repeat this sentence 10 times very slowly while picturing your body at your ideal weight.

Step Three: Say, "I am able to move toward my ideal weight with increasing comfort." Repeat this statement 10 times while picturing yourself looking and feeling more comfortable.

Step Four: Say, "I *am* able to move toward higher levels of wellness and positive energy." Repeat this statement slowly five times while visualizing yourself moving to increased states of wellness and becoming filled with positive energy.

Step Five: Slowly open your eyes and prepare to eat, carrying with you the image of yourself at your ideal weight.

- Although most chains have converted to all-vegetable fat for frying, fried foods still are among the highest in fat and calories.
- Take a trip to the salad bar for a lower fat sidedish alternative to fries and onion rings. Keep your salad lean by going easy on the bacon bits, croutons, regular salad dressing, and prepared salads, and by choosing low calorie or yogurt-based dressings.

Plan Ahead

- Make up for the extra calories and possible lack of variety in the meal you eat out by having lower calorie, nutrient-rich foods at home. Low or nonfat dairy products, fresh fruits and vegetables, and high fiber breads and cereals provide a lot of the nutrients in shorter supply in meals away from home.
- Healthy choices for snacks at home that you can prepare ahead of time include pita wedges with a cottage cheese and vegetable dip, high fiber muffins, a low fat yogurt parfait made with fruit and dry cereal, or a mixed fruit cup.

Eating on the Road

- Feel like you and your family live in the car? Be sure to take along individu-ally portioned juices, raw vegetables, low fat cheese or peanut butter and whole grain crackers, snack boxes or bags of dried fruits, and seasoned, air-popped popcorn.

- Your best breakfast bets on the road are cereal with milk, waffles or pancakes with fresh fruit toppings, a bagel or toast with preserves, fruits, and juices.
- If you are at a convention, buffet, or party, fill up first on raw vegetables and seltzer. Then survey the scene to decide what else to eat.
- Watch out for foods that sound healthier than they are: teriyaki dishes are low in fat but high in sodium, potato skins often are fried and with high fat toppings, pasta primavera can be made with cream, and light menu items may be nothing more than high-fat appetizers.

RECOMMENDING FOODS AND SUPPLEMENTS TO CLIENTS

Use Table 9.4, Client Nutritional Prescriptions, when recommending foods and supplements to clients.

Table 9.4   Client Nutritional Prescriptions

Condition	Nutritional Prescription
Acidosis[a]	Eat small amounts of citrus fruits, gradually increasing the amount; eat more apricots, avocados, corn, dates, uncooked fruits, grapes, honey, kelp, lemons, maple syrup, millet, molasses, oranges, raisins, figs, uncooked vegetables, and melons (alone)
AIDS/HIV	Make the diet 75% fresh and uncooked fruits and vegetables; drink 10 ounces of juiced kale, spinach, beet greens, carrots, beet root, garlic and onions; eat unripened papaya and fresh pineapple for digestive enzymes; eliminate diet and regular colas, and other junk and processed foods, including anything containing caffeine; alternate psyllium husks with freshly ground flaxseeds (put 1 teaspoon in a glass of water and drink down immediately); test for food sensitivities with muscle or pulse testing and eliminate anything that tests "weak"; daily in addition to a good multivitamin and multimineral tablet, take selenium, chromium, coenzyme Q_{10}, B complex, vitamin C, copper, and vitamin A.
Allergies	Avoid all sugars, wheat, salt, flours, coffee and alcohol; drink as much citrus water as possible every day (squeeze the following in 1 gallon of water: 10 lemons, 2 oranges, and 2 grapefruit); drink 1 tablespoon cider vinegar and 1 tablespoon honey in water at least 3 times a day; take up to 5 grams a day of vitamin C, a balanced B complex, vitamin E (up to 800 IU daily), 1 tablespoon crude pollen a day; take digestive enzymes after every meal; test for food sensitivities and avoid those foods you are sensitive to
Alzheimer's	Take a daily multivitamin and multimineral and additional vitamins D, E, A, B complex, zinc, selenium, carnitine, choline, coenzyme Q_{10}, lecithin,

Table 9.4 *(continued)*

Condition	Nutritional Prescription
	Pycnogenol or grape seed extract, garlic, kelp, vitamin C, and calcium/magnesium; take 2 tablespoons apple pectin daily to excrete aluminum (from unfiltered drinking water, antacids, dental amalgams, and cooking utensils) and other toxic minerals
Appetite (poor)	Use a high-potency multivitamin and mineral complex daily; take 100 mg or more vitamin B complex daily before meals (use sublingual form if possible); take 80 mg zinc (plus 3 mg copper to balance zinc) daily; start with 1/2 teaspoon of Brewer's yeast and work up to 1 tablespoon daily; drink 3 or more cups of skim milk, soymilk, Rice Dream, almond milk, soy carob drink, or yogurt fruit shakes daily; use cream soups made with soymilk; between meals snack on avocados, banana soy pudding, nuts and nut butters, buttermilk, cheese, chicken or tuna, custard, and yogurt; avoid drinking liquids before or during meals; try six small meals rather than 3 large ones.
Arteriosclerosis	Eat a high-fiber, low-fat diet with fruits, vegetables, and grains as main foods, especially dark green leafy vegetables, legumes, nuts, seeds, soybeans, wheat germ, and whole grains; use small amounts of olive oil on salads and unheated with steamed vegetables; avoid chips, candy, fried foods, gravies, pies, cakes, sweet rolls or desserts, processed canned or baked goods, red meat, margarine and butter or its substitutes, ice cream, salt and all foods containing white flour and/or sugar, coffee, colas, alcohol, and highly spiced food; take 1500 mg calcium/magnesium daily (at least partly at bedtime), 100 mg coenzyme Q_{10} daily, flaxseed oil as per label, garlic capsules as per label, 25,000 IU vitamin A, 200 IU vitamin E/day and work up to 1,000 IU/day, 5,000–20,000 mg buffered vitamin C/day in divided doses, lecithin granules or capsules as directed on label to break down and expel fat, digestive enzymes to destroy free radicals and improve digestion, Pycnogenol or grape seed extract as per label to enhance heart tissue, 100 mg 3x/day vitamin B complex to dilate small arteries and assist relaxation.
Arthritis	Focus meals around whole grains, fresh vegetables and fruits, eliminating sugar (doughnuts, cakes, pies, candy, etc.), milk and dairy products, red meat, caffeine, salt, and tobacco; eat more fish, especially herring, salmon, and tuna; avoid foods from the nightshade family (tomatoes, potatoes, eggplant, peppers, paprika, and cayenne for one month (if no relief, reintroduce them slowly to see if they affect symptoms); test for sensitivity to wheat and corn; drink two cups of fresh grapefruit juice daily in the a.m.; drink 10 ounces fresh carrot juice mixed with 6 ounces fresh spinach and 10 ounces of carrot juice mixed with 6 ounces celery juice, after noon, spaced at least 2 hours apart; avoid Aspartame (artificial sweetener); eat more sulphur-containing foods (needed to repair bone, cartilage, and connective tissue and aid in calcium absorption): asparagus, eggs, garlic, onions; consume green leafy vegetables (vitamin K), rice (contains histi-

(continued)

Table 9.4   *(continued)*

Condition	Nutritional Prescription
	dine that removes the excess levels of copper and iron in many arthritis sufferers), eat fresh pineapple frequently (contains bromelain, an enzyme that reduces inflammation); eat some form of fiber (ground flaxseeds, oat, or rice bran) every day; take chelated calcium (2,000 mg daily) with magnesium (1,000 mg daily), copper (3 mg daily), zinc (50 mg daily), and boron (3 mg daily) to prevent bone loss and strengthen connective tissue; take an additional B complex vitamin daily (to reduce swelling), vitamin C (3,000–10,000 mg) + 500 mg bioflavonoids and Pycnogenol (as directed on label) daily (for pain and inflammation), vitamin E (400 IU daily) to protect the joints and increase joint mobility, and cayenne capsules to relieve pain
Asthma	Eat mostly fresh fruits and vegetables, nuts and seeds, oatmeal, brown rice, and whole grains (if not sensitive), garlic and onions (contain quercetin and mustard oils that fight inflammation), have a green drink at least daily (blend spinach, celery, beet greens, endive or romaine lettuce, parsley, and unsweetened pineapple juice)
Back Pain	10 ounces fresh carrot juice mixed with 6 ounces fresh spinach juice daily after noon or carrot juice with a little fresh beet and apple juice; eat at least 1 large green salad daily; eat less protein; avoid eating after 6 p.m.
Blood Pressure (high)	Take a daily multivitamin and multimineral; test for food sensitivities and avoid identified foods; avoid caffeine, meat, cheese, sugar, sour cream, alcohol, tobacco, salt (if salt sensitive), artificial sweeteners; eat more fresh vegetables and bananas, apricots, peaches, and prunes; take: 2 garlic capsules 3x/day, carnitine up to 1,000 mg 3–4x/day, coenzyme Q_{10} up to 30 mg 3x/day, 2 teaspoons or 3–6 capsules of flaxseed and/or borage oil, vitamin E (start with 100 IU and build up to 400 IU daily over a few months), vitamin B complex (100 mg 2x/day with meals), lecithin (1 teaspoon 3x/day before meals to emulsify fat and lower blood pressure), vitamin C (3,000 to 6,000 mg/day in divided doses)
Breast Cancer	Prevention of or treatment for diagnosed cases: Eat organic fresh fruits and vegetables (especially broccoli, Brussels sprouts, cabbage, cauliflower, carrots, pumpkin, squash, sweet potatoes, yams, fresh apples, cherries, grapes, plums, and all types of berries, whole grains, legumes (dried beans and peas), raw nuts (except peanuts) and seeds, and soured (unsweetened) products (such as yogurt), garlic and onions; take extra wheat or rice bran (to keep toxic wastes from being absorbed; take this separately from supplements); limit but not completely, soy products (contain enzyme inhibitors); avoid completely alcohol, caffeine, junk foods, processed refined foods, saturated fat, salt, sugar or white flour or pasta (unless whole wheat), meat or dairy products (many animals treated with hormones), any supplements containing iron (promotes tumor growth); take the following supplements: beta-carotene (10,000 IU daily), coenzyme Q_{10}, essential fatty acids (boarge, black currant seed, or flaxseed oil), selenium (200–400

Table 9.4 *(continued)*

Condition	Nutritional Prescription
	mcg daily), vitamin A (50,000 IU daily)[b], vitamin B complex (100 mg daily), choline (100 mg 3x/day aids in reducing estrogen production), vitamin C with bioflavonoids (5,000–20,000 mg daily in divided doses), vitamin E in emulsion (start with 400 IU daily; increase slowly to 1,000 IU daily to aid in hormone and immune function)
Bronchitis	Include garlic (natural antibiotic) and onions (contain the anti-inflammatory quercetin) in the daily diet; drink pure water, herbal teas and soups; avoid mucus-forming foods (dairy products, sugar, sweet fruits, and white flour products, processed foods); avoid gas-producing foods (cabbage, cauliflower, and beans); eat a vegetarian diet; have a green drink daily (blend spinach, celery, beet greens, endive or romaine lettuce with unsweetened pineapple juice); take the following supplements: vitamin A (20,000 IU twice daily for a month, then reduce to 15,000 IU[b]), vitamin C with bioflavonoids (3,000–10,000 mg daily in divided doses), vitamin E (400 IU or more twice a day with at least 100 mg vitamin C), coenzyme Q_{10} calcium (1,000 mg) with magnesium (500 mg) in asporotate or chelated form, and a daily multivitamin and multimineral
Cancer	Drink 1 pint of fresh juice combining 3 ounces fresh beet, 10 ounces fresh carrot, asparagus, or cabbage juice daily after noon; drink 1–2 cups of fresh grape, black cherry, or apple juice in the morning daily; eat lots of fresh and cooked onions and garlic (detoxifies carcinogens); include whole grains, nuts, especially almonds, seeds, brown rice, millet, oatmeal, cruciferous vegetables (broccoli, cauliflower, and cabbage help a precursor to estrogen break up into a benign rather than a cancer-causing form), brussels sprouts, cantaloupe, carrots, pumpkin, squash, yams, apples, berries, chickpeas, lentils, red beans, plums, citrus fruits (prevent cancer-causing hormones from latching onto cells), hot peppers (keeps toxic molecules from attaching to cells), soybeans (prevent growth of new blood vessels to cancer cells), tomatoes (disrupt the union of cells that produce carcinogens); avoid processed foods (white bread, pies, cakes, candy, canned foods), luncheon meats, hot dogs, smoked or cured meats, other meats, salt, sugar, alcohol, coffee and tea (except herbal teas); in addition to a daily multivitamin and multimineral, take 10,000 I.U. vitamin A, 100 mg coenzyme Q_{10}, 200 mcg selenium, 5,000–10,000 mg vitamin C with bioflavonoids
Common Cold	Stop eating solid foods; drink citrus water (squeeze 10 lemons, 2 oranges, and 2 grapefruit, add to a gallon of filtered water and sip throughout the day; 2 capsules or 1 clove of fresh garlic 4x/day; 1 gram vitamin C every 2 hours
Cystitis (bladder infection)	For Prevention: Drink at least six 8-ounce glasses of water daily; drink 10 ounces fresh carrot juice combined with 3 ounces each beet and cucumber juice (after noon), and then 10 ounces carrot juice combined with 6 ounces fresh spinach juice at least 2 hours later; During an infection:

(continued)

Table 9.4 *(continued)*

Condition	Nutritional Prescription
	Include the natural diuretics, celery, parsley, and watermelon in the diet; avoid taking iron supplements (including in multivitamins) until healed (bacteria require iron for growth); in addition to daily supplements, take: 500 mg buffered vitamin C every 4 hours for duration of infection (then cut down to 1,000 to 5,000 mg daily for maintenance), 1 g bioflavonoids daily, 25,000 IU vitamin A during the infection[b], and 50 mg zinc every day
Depression	Muscle or pulse test anything eaten; eat a diet based on raw fruits and vegetables, Soy products, brown rice, millet, and dried beans and peas (without these complex carbohydrates, serotonin is depleted and anxiety and depression can result); eat salmon and whitefish to increase alertness; to lift spirits, eat turkey and salmon; omit wheat bread, noodles, pasta, pies, cakes, cookies, and anything else that has wheat in it (read labels carefully: wheat gluten has been linked to depression); avoid artificial sweeteners and anything containing the amino acid phenylalanine; avoid saturated fats (meat or fried foods lead to sluggishness, slow thinking, and fatigue by interfering with blood flow to the brain); avoid all sweets (the increase in energy is quickly followed by fatigue and depression); avoid alcohol, caffeine, and processed foods; every day take: a good multivitamin and multimineral (to correct deficiencies often associated with depression), 2,000–5,000 mg vitamin C plus rutin (prevents depression), up to 50 mg per pound of body weight of L-Tyrosine[c] with 50 mg vitamin B_6 and 1000 mg vitamin C for better absorption, vitamin B Complex (necessary for normal brain and nervous system functioning: take as an injection for serious depression and only under health care practitioner's supervision), lecithin (for brain function as directed on label[d], calcium and magnesium chelate or asporotate (1,500–2,000 mg/day: 1,000 mg/day calms the nervous system), essential fatty acids, black currant seed oil or primrose oil (as directed on label) at meals to aid in the transmission of nerve impulses
Digestion/ Indigestion	Have a green drink at least 3 times a week (spinach, celery, beet greens, endive, parsley mixed with unsweetened pineapple juice) and chew each mouthful well; focus on greens, fresh fruits, garlic, onions, potatoes, papaya, pineapple, and nonfat yogurt with active cultures; eat simple meals and each day have a large bowl of steamed zucchini and/or green beans, and/or asparagus, yams (nourishing and easy to digest), and/or potatoes; drink 2–6 ounces of aloe vera juice daily and two cups of fenugreek tea
Dermatitis	Add brown rice and millet to the diet; avoid all dairy products, sugar, white flour, fried and processed foods and fats; try a gluten-free diet for 2 weeks (find gluten-free products at health food stores and read labels and avoid any foods that contain barley, oats, rye, or wheat, hydrolyzed vegetable protein, textured vegetable protein, hydrolyzed plant protein,

Table 9.4 *(continued)*

Condition	Nutritional Prescription
	malt, modified food starch, most soy sauces, grain vinegars, binders, fillers, excipients and "natural flavorings," hot dogs, gravies, luncheon meat, beer, mustard, ketchup, nondairy creamer, white vinegar, curry powder, or seasonings); avoid egg nog or any foods containing raw egg; in addition to daily multivitamin and multimineral, take: vitamin B complex 50–100 mg 3x/day with meals
Gall Bladder (distress, bloating, gas, nausea, after fatty meal, or sharp pain in upper right abdomen)	Focus meals around fresh fruits and vegetables and grains (if not sensitive); avoid fatty and fried foods; increase fiber with whole grains, fresh fruits, and vegetables; use muscle testing to eliminate possible food sensitivities; for breakfast for 3 weeks: blend either 2 oranges or 2 small apples with 1 clove of fresh garlic, 1 tablespoon of olive oil, and the juice of 2 fresh lemons; follow with 2 glasses of warm herb tea or distilled water; nothing solid until lunch; lunch: eat either all fruit or all vegetable meals (the latter with 2 tablespoons of sesame butter); dinner: steam or bake potatoes, yams, squash, or have soup or vegetable casseroles with steamed greens and a salad and one slice of whole grain bread (every other night); at both lunch and dinner, have 2 tablespoons of grated beets with 1 tablespoon of olive oil and 1 teaspoon of fresh lemon juice; for stones: the first night drink a mixture of 2 ounces of fresh lemon juice and 2 ounces of olive oil; the second night increase both to 4 ounces each; drink 6–8 glasses of water daily; in addition to regular supplements, take 500 mg lecithin 3 times a day (helps bile keep cholesterol in solution and prevent stones)
Gout	Eliminate foods that promote uric acid (meat, gravies, rich foods such as cakes and pies, white flour and sugar products, dried beans, cauliflower, fish, lentils, oatmeal, peas, poultry, spinach, and anything containing yeast); avoid purine-rich foods (anchovies, asparagus, consomme, herring, meat gravies and broths, mushrooms, mussels, all organ meats, sardines, sweetbreads); lose weight gradually if overweight; increase fresh fruit and vegetable consumption; drink 7 ounces of fresh carrot juice combined with 4 ounces fresh celery, 2 ounces fresh parsley, and 3 ounces fresh spinach juice daily after noon and/or drink 10 ounces fresh carrot juice combined with 6 ounces spinach juice (at least 2 hours apart); drink 3 quarts of liquid daily; eliminate all alcohol drinks; eat one-half pound of cherries or strawberries daily to neutralize uric acid; eliminate vitamin A intake if attacks continue
Fibrocystic breasts	Eat a low-fat, high-fiber diet, including more raw fruits, vegetables, nuts and seeds, whole grains, and (dried) beans; avoid coffee, tea (except herbals), cola drinks or chocolate, alcohol, meat and animal fats, cooking oils (use olive oil for cooking and salads), fried foods, sugar (in any form), tobacco, and all white flour products; take vitamin E (400–600 IU daily), kelp (divided daily doses of 1,500–2,000 mg to provide iodine that is often deficient in this condition), 15,000 IU daily (10,000 if preg-

(continued)

Table 9.4 *(continued)*

Condition	Nutritional Prescription
	nant) vitamin A, 50 mg vitamin B complex 3x/day, vitamin C (divided doses of 2,000–4,000 mg daily), proteolytic enzymes with bromelain to reduce inflammation and soreness (as per label)
Fibromy-algia	Test for food sensitivities, then eat 4–5 small meals a day of 50% raw foods and fresh juices and combine with the following if not sensitive to: millet, brown rice, raw nuts and seeds, deepwater fish, skinless turkey or chicken; drink at least 8 glasses of distilled water; avoid tomatoes, green peppers, potatoes, and eggplant if associated with muscle pain and discomfort; avoid saturated fats, including meat and dairy products; avoid caffeine, alcohol, sugars, fried foods, shellfish, white flour products such as pasta and bread, any wheat and brewer's yeast; muscle test and use the following as appropriate: a multivitamin and multimineral daily, coenzyme Q_{10}, lecithin, malic acid and magnesium, manganese, digestive enzymes, vitamin A, vitamin C with bioflavonoids, vitamin E, vitamin B complex, primrose or black currant or flaxseed oil, and grape seed extract as directed on label; also take 6 capsules of garlic per day in divided doses with meals, and 2,000 mg per day of calcium/magnesium (to relieve muscle spasms and pain)
Headache	Test for food allergies, then try eliminating foods containing tyramine, phenylalanine (aspartame, Equal, NutraSweet), monosodium glutamate/MSG, hot dogs, luncheon meats. alcohol, bananas, cheese, chicken, chocolate, citrus fruits, cold cuts, herring, onions, peanut butter, pork, smoked fish, sour cream, vinegar, wine, and fresh-baked yeast products, chewing gum, ice cream, ice cold beverages, salt; eat small and frequent meals to stabilize blood sugar; eat more almonds, almond milk, parsley, fennel, watercress, cherries, pineapple, and garlic
Heart attack	Eat foods high in fiber, almonds, Brewer's yeast, sesame seeds, kelp and sea vegetables; avoid red meat, spicy foods, salt, sugar, white flour foods, refined sugars (candy, cakes, pies, cookies, etc.), coffee, black tea, colas, chocolate, and alcohol; take: choline and inositol as per label to remove fat from liver and bloodstream, coenzyme Q_{10} 100 mg 3x/day, work up to 800 mg/day, vitamin E unless on anticoagulant then discuss with health care provider, 200 mcg selenium, grape seed extract 150–300 mg/day (powerful antioxidant), 1500 mg calcium/day in divided doses to help maintain proper heart rhythm and blood pressure, chromium 100 mcg daily to increase "good cholesterol," primrose or salmon oil to protect heart muscle, 6 capsules garlic to promote circulation, proteolytic enzymes as per label to reduce inflammation and prevent damage to arteries, vitamin A as per label, to mg zinc/day with 3 mg copper/day, vitamin B complex daily, Pycnogenol as per label to strengthen connective heart tissue, vitamin C 3,000–6,000 mg/day to prevent blood clots and aid in thinning the blood, L-Carnitine 500 mg twice daily on empty stomach with vitamins B complex and C for better absorption, 1,000 mg taurine

Table 9.4   *(continued)*

Condition	Nutritional Prescription
	daily to stabilize heartbeat, 100 mg potassium daily to balance electrolytes if taking blood pressure medication or cortisone, vitamin E up to 1,000 IU while under medical supervision
Heart Failure (Congestive)	Follow a low-fat, high-fiber, vegetarian diet (see arteriosclerosis); take the following supplements: coenzyme Q_{10} 10–30 mg 2–3x/day, magnesium 400–800 mg a day, vitamin C 1,000–4,000 mg daily in divided doses, selenium 200 mcg/day, vitamin B complex 50 mg/day, taurine up to 3,000 mg/day, vitamin E work up to 800 mg/day
Heartburn/ Hiatal	Eat small, frequent meals and allow 3 hrs between last food or fluid and sleep; eat low-fat foods (fatty foods increase stomach acid); avoid antacids; drink 7 ounces of fresh carrot juice combined with 4 ounces fresh celery, 2 ounces fresh parsley, and 3 ounces fresh spinach juice after noon, daily; avoid coffee, tea, chocolate, alcohol, citrus fruits and juices, onions, tomatoes, and any food or drug that irritates; take 1–2 acidophillus capsules to relieve heartburn
Hemorrhoids	Shift to a diet centered around fresh fruits and vegetables, whole grains, and dried beans; take 1–2 tablespoons of linseed oil daily to soften stools; drink 8 ounces fresh carrot juice mixed with 4 ounces fresh spinach juice, 2 ounces fresh turnip, and 2 ounces watercress daily after noon; eat more kale and dark green leafy vegetables to enhance vitamin K that treats bleeding hemorrhoids; drink 1 teaspoon psyllium powder or seeds in water
Herpes	Eat whole foods; take a lysine supplement (1,000 mgs 3x/day at the initial signs of infection; 500–1,000 mg/day for maintenance; take on an empty stomach with water or juice and take no longer than 6 months at a time; avoid: sugar, caffeine, trans-fatty acids (margarine and other partially-hydrogenated oils), foods high in arginine that are beneficial to the herpes virus (peanuts, dried beans, cashews, coconut, wheat bran, chocolate, cottonseed oil, corn, oats, dairy products, meat, barley); take: vitamin A 50,000 IU daily[b], vitamin B complex 50 mg and up 3x/day, vitamin C with bioflavonoids 5,000–10,000 mg/day, Zinc 50–100 mg daily in divided doses, acidophillus 3x/day as per label, lecithin as per label, 3 garlic tablets 3x/day with meals, 600 IU vitamin E emulsion, 1500 mg calcium with magnesium daily, multivitamin and multimineral tablet daily, digestive enzyme; test for sensitivity to foods, especially citrus fruits and avoid those that test negative
Hypogly-cemia	Test for food sensitivities and avoid any negative results; eat large amounts of raw and lightly steamed broccoli, carrots, Jerusalem artichokes, raw spinach, squash, and string beans; eat beans, brown rice, potatoes, soy products, lentils, apples, bananas, avocados, cantaloupes, persimmons, lemons, and grapefruit; for protein eat fish, grains, seeds, skinless white

(continued)

Table 9.4   *(continued)*

Condition	Nutritional Prescription
	turkey or white chicken breast, low-fat yogurt; avoid corn, hominy, noo-dles, pasta, white rice, yams, bacon, fried foods, cold cuts, gravies, ham, sausage, dairy products (except yogurt, kefir, and buttermilk), caffeine, alcohol and tobacco, anything with sugar in it, sweet fruits, grape or prune juice or mix it half and half with water before drinking, artificial colors or preservatives; eat 6 to 8 small meals and a small snack before bedtime if well-tolerated; for a low-blood-sugar reaction, carry crackers and cheese or peanut butter; in addition to a daily multivitamin and multimineral, test for, then take the following supplements: 200–600 mcg chromium picolinate and spirulina daily to stabilize blood sugar, digestive enzymes[d], 50–150 mg vitamin B complex daily, 50 mg zinc to help release insulin, 400 IU or more of vitamin E to improve energy level and circulation, 3,000–8,000 mg vitamin C daily in divided doses to enhance adrenal function, 1,000 mg L-glutamine daily with water or juice on an empty stomach to reduce sugar cravings, L-cysteine daily as per label to keep blood sugar stable, L-Carnitine daily as per label to convert body fat to energy, 1/2 teaspoon psyllium husks or powder in a glass of water daily to keep the colon clean and slow down blood sugar reactions
Kidney stones (Due to calcium oxalate or uric acid crystals in the urine)	Drink at least 8 glasses of filtered water daily; after noon, drink 9 ounces of fresh carrot combined with 5 ounces of fresh celery and 2 ounces of fresh parsley juice; eat foods rich in magnesium (barley, corn, bran, buckwheat, rye, oats, brown rice, potatoes, and bananas), watermelon (diuretic and cleanser), cranberry juice (to acidify the urine); avoid the amino acid L-cysteine (crystallizes stones) and oxalic acid-containing or -producing foods (asparagus, beets, parsley, rhubarb, sorrel, spinach, Swiss chard, vegetables of the cabbage family) as well as alcohol, caffeine (tea, coffee, chocolate, colas), dried figs, lamb, nuts, pepper and poppy seeds; after meals take 1/2 teaspoon cream of tartar in 1/2 cup of water for 4 days; avoid: salt, naturally carbonated and mineral waters (high in calcium content); reduce intake of animal proteins (meat, milk, yogurt, ice cream, cream, chicken, fish) to no more than 3 ounces at lunch and dinner (animal protein results in excess calcium in the urine); test for, then take: up to 50 mg/day of vitamin B[6] and up to 400 mg/day of magnesium to lower urinary oxalates and help prevent recurrences; apply castor oil pack on the abdomen or back for pain during an acute attack
Liver Conditions	Avoid: all meats except fish and chicken, sugar, alcohol, commercial coffee or tea, fried foods, processed foods or flours, salt, strong spices, preservatives, additives or synthetic vitamins, all canned foods except asparagus; eat more globe artichokes (protects the liver); drink green drinks, carrot juice and beet juice (See "bronchitis"); *Liver Flush Drink*: For 3 weeks drink the following for breakfast: the juice of 2 oranges, or 2 small apples, blended with 1 clove fresh garlic (or 1/2 teaspoon raw grated ginger root), 1 tablespoon olive oil, and the juice of two lemons;

Table 9.4   *(continued)*

Condition	Nutritional Prescription
	follow immediately with two glasses of warm liquid, preferably distilled water or dandelion or parsley tea; avoid eating any solids until lunch; lunch: either fresh fruit or vegetable meals including globe artichoke (protects the liver); the first and third week have 2 tablespoons of sesame butter with any vegetable meal; every day have 2 tablespoons grated beets plus 1 tablespoon olive oil and 1/2 tablespoon fresh lemon juice; each night before bed, drink 2 cups of strong yarrow, dandelion, and parsley tea; *Optional*: the first night of the third week, drink a mix of 2 ounces of olive oil and 2 ounces of lemon juice; the second night, increase to 4 ounces each; dinner: steamed or baked potatoes, yams, squashes, fresh soups, and casseroles, with steamed vegetables and dark green salad and 2 tablespoons of grated beets plus 1 tablespoon olive oil and 1/2 teaspoon fresh lemon juice; after assessing for sensitivities, take 1,200 mg lecithin capsules 3x/day before meals (to protect liver cells), vitamin B complex as per label (essential for normal liver function), primrose or salmon oil as per label (essential fatty acids combat liver inflammation); also: apply warm castor oil packs over liver (left upper abdomen) for 1/2 to 2 hours and keep it warm with a heating pad
Memory loss	Test for food sensitivities, then eat a diet high in raw foods, Brewer's yeast, brown rice, farm eggs, nuts, soybeans, wheat germ, legumes, and millet; avoid dairy products and wheat for at least one month to see if there is memory improvement; avoid candy, cake, pies, doughnuts, and all refined sugar that "turn off" the brain; avoid junk foods and fried foods; take the following supplements: a daily multivitamin and multimineral, lecithin granules or capsules to improve brain function, 100 mg vitamin B complex, 3,000–10,000 mg vitamin C daily in divided doses, gradually increase intake of vitamin E from 400 IU daily to 1,200 IU to improve blood flow to the brain, 50–80 mg zinc daily to remove toxic substances from the brain; take amino acids L-Glutamine plus L-aspartic acid on an empty stomach with water or juice to enhance brain function
Meniere's Disease	Try a hypoglycemic regime; *see* hypoglycemia
Menopause	Test for food sensitivities, then eat 50% raw foods, and more white fish, sardines, salmon with bones, blackstrap molasses, broccoli, dandelion greens, and kelp; eat more phytoestrogenic foods: soybeans, soymilk, tofu, miso, flaxseeds, pomegranates, and dates; avoid dairy products and meat (they trigger hot flashes and leech calcium from bones), sugar, alcohol, caffeine, spicy foods, and hot soups and drink (they trigger hot flashes, and aggravate mood swings and urinary incontinence), salt (increases urinary excretion of calcium); daily, take a multivitamin and multimineral; test for, then take those testing positive: lecithin (1200 mg

(continued)

Table 9.4   *(continued)*

Condition	Nutritional Prescription
	3x/day) and vitamin E (400–1,600 IU daily), vitamin C (3,000–10,000 mg daily), primrose or black currant seed oil (per label) to reduce hot flashes, 99 mg potassium daily to replace potassium lost through perspiration during hot flashes, vitamin B complex (per label) to enhance circulation, cellular function, and mood, 2,000 mg calcium with magnesium, boron, and silica daily to relieve nervousness and irritability and protect against bone loss
Menstrual Bleeding (Excessive)	Test for food sensitivities; take a daily multivitamin and multimineral that contain at least 400 mg of magnesium to aid in the metabolism of fatty acids (see borage and flaxseed oil recommendation below; eat grapefruit, especially the white pulp containing bioflavonoids; eat the following high vitamin K vegetables to prevent abnormal bleeding: broccoli, brussels sprouts, spinach, and cabbage; avoid processed and partially hydrogenated vegetable oils, alcohol, sugars/sweets, nicotine, caffeine, and any foods testing "weak"; follow the Liver Flush periodically (*see* Liver Conditions); take the following vitamins and supplements: 75,000 vitamin A[b] for several months tapering down to no more than 25,000 IU daily, 400 IU daily vitamin E, 15–30 mg zinc daily, vitamin C with bioflavonoids in 3 divided doses/day, 1–2 teaspoons a day of flaxseed oil or 200–300 mg/day of borage oil capsules (essential fatty acids may reduce excessive bleeding)
Migraine	Test for food sensitivities and avoid any that test "weak"; some common foods known to precipitate attacks are chocolate; citrus fruits; aged, pickled, soured, yeasty, or fermented foods; alcohol, especially red wine; adopt a dietary regime low in sugars and high in protein (migraine is associated with low blood sugar) and eat more almonds, almond milk, watercress, parsley, garlic, cherries, fennel, and fresh pineapple; avoid avocados, bananas, eggplant, hard cheese, red plums, tomatoes, raspberries, cabbage, canned fish, dairy products, aspirin, spicy foods, salt, fried foods and fatty and greasy foods, acid-forming foods (cereal, bread, grains, including pasta), and anything with monosodium glutamate (MSG) or nitrites (hot dogs and luncheon meats primarily) in it; take a hypoallergenic multivitamin and multimineral; take additional chelated calcium (2,000 mg) and magnesium (1,000 mg) daily to enhance muscular relaxation and nerve impulse transmission, 60 mg coenzyme Q_{10} daily to increase brain blood flow, 2 capsules of garlic 3x/day to detoxify the body and brain, vitamin B complex (per label), 3,000–6,000 mg vitamin C daily
Mitral Valve Prolapse	Test for food sensitivities, then follow diet for hypoglycemia (*see* hypoglycemia); avoid chocolate, sugar, caffeine, and other stimulants; to lessen or eliminate the need for beta blocking drugs, take a multivitamin and multimineral daily, 10–30 mgm coenzyme Q_{10} daily, vitamin B_6 daily, 800 mg magnesium daily, 250 to 1,000 mg carnitine 3x/day

Table 9.4 *(continued)*

Condition	Nutritional Prescription
Multiple Sclerosis	Test for food sensitivities, then eat a diet low in saturated fat; a vegetarian regime is the best treatment; eat only organically grown food including eggs, fruits, gluten-free grains, vegetables (especially dark leafy greens that supply vitamin K), raw nuts and seeds, and cold-pressed oils; avoid alcohol, chocolate, coffee, dairy products, fried foods, alcohol, salt, spices, sugar, tobacco, meat, highly seasoned foods, and wheat; use Liver Flush drink periodically (*see* liver); take a fiber supplement to avoid constipation; take coenzyme 90 mg Q_{10} daily, 2 capsules of garlic 3x/day to protect against toxic substances, 100 mg vitamin B complex daily to maintain a healthy nervous system, lecithin to protect the myelin sheaths (per label), 1 teaspoon acidophilus 2x/day on an empty stomach to help detoxify the body and enhance absorption, grape seed extract (per label) to reduce inflammation, 300–1,000 mg potassium/day to enhance muscle function, 2,000–3,000 mg/day of calcium (with 1,000–1,500 mg/day of magnesium and 800 IU vitamin D daily to enhance its absorption), and 5–10 mg manganese/day (often deficient in individuals diagnosed with MS), 3,000–5,000 mg buffered vitamin C to promote production of antiviral protein interferon; alternate 30 mg zinc and 2 mg copper every other day with 500 mg N-acetylcysteine; daily take borage oil capsules (up to 500 mg/day) and 3,000 mg/day of fish oil capsules
Osteoporosis	Test for food sensitivities, then eat foods high in calcium and vitamin D (broccoli, chestnuts, clams, dandelion greens, dark green leafy vegetables, flounder, hazelnuts, kale, kelp, molasses, oats, oysters, salmon, sardines with their bones, sea vegetables, sesame [seeds, and tahini], shrimp, turnip greens, and wheatgerm soybeans [tempeh, tofu, soy milk], turnip greens, and wheat germ); eat foods high in sulfur to aid in healthy bones: garlic and onions; limit intake of foods high in oxalic acid that inhibit absorption of calcium: almonds, asparagus, beet greens, cashews, chard, rhubarb, and spinach; avoid substances that inhibit calcium uptake: yeast products (high in phosphorus and competes with calcium), caffeine, carbonated soft drinks, animal products (meat, milk, poultry, fish, eggs, and cheese), alcohol, citrus fruits, tomatoes, tobacco, sugar, salt, aluminum-containing antacids, or foods cooked in aluminum containers; take a multivitamin and multimineral daily and 1,500–2,0000 mg calcium (with 3 mg boron, 3 mg copper, silica as directed on the label, 400 IU vitamins E and D, digestive enzymes with betaine hydrochloride, L-lysine (on an empty stomach with water or juice only as directed on label), 50 mg zinc, and 1,000 mg magnesium to enhance calcium absorption), 3 mg copper daily to aid in bone formation; also helpful: kelp, cod liver oil (vitamins A and D), vitamin C (3,000 mg and up)

(continued)

Table 9.4   *(continued)*

Condition	Nutritional Prescription
Palpitations	Eat whole foods, emphasizing fresh produce, magnesium-rich foods (raw nuts, whole grains, soybeans, fresh peas, wheat germ, swiss chard, figs, citrus fruits, dark green leafy vegetables), and potassium-rich foods (bananas, fresh vegetable juices, raw cabbage, turkey, apples, baked potato, wheat germ, spinach, dried fruit, fresh fruit and vegetables of all kinds); avoid coffee, tea, soft drinks, and chocolate; test for, then take: 400 IU vitamin E daily, 50 mg vitamin B complex daily, up to 1,000 mg vitamin C with bioflavonoids 3x/day, 800 mg magnesium a day, and 300 to 1,000 mg carnitine 3x/day to normalize heart rhythm
Parkinson's	Test for food sensitivities first, then eat a diet high in fiber to ward off constipation (fresh fruits and vegetables); put a teaspoon of psyllium seed in half a glass of water and drink immediately or eat reconstituted prunes and figs for breakfast; eat foods high in vitamins C and E that seem to delay the progression of the disease; take a multivitamin and multimineral daily and gradually increase vitamin E to 2,000 IU daily and vitamin C to 3,000 mg daily
PMS	Test for food sensitivities first, then eat primarily fresh fruits, raw nuts, vegetables, fish, eggs, wheat germ, and whole grains to insure adequate zinc, essential fatty acids, and vitamin C to reduce inflammation-producing prostaglandins; avoid partially-hydrogenated oils found in cakes, cookies, and chips (they imbalance prostaglandins that increase PMS), dairy products, sugar and refined carbohydrates, caffeine and nonorganic meats that stress the adrenals (underlying PMS); take a daily multivitamin and multimineral and additional B complex; to heal the tired adrenals underlying PMS: take 400–1,000 vitamin C and 400 IU vitamin E daily
Prostate Hypertrophy	Test for food sensitivities; follow a low-fat diet, avoiding margarine, hydrogenated vegetable oils, and fried foods (they interfere with prostaglandin metabolism); drink 10 ounces of fresh carrot juice combined with 3 ounces each of beet and cucumber or 10 ounces fresh carrot juice and 6 ounces spinach, and/or 8 ounces carrot, 4 ounces asparagus, and 4 ounces dark green lettuce; eat 1 ounce pumpkin seeds or take pumpkin seed oil capsules as per label daily (zinc tends to shrink the prostate); avoid alcohol; take a multivitamin and multimineral; the amino acids glycine, alanine, and glutamic acid are also useful
Secondhand Smoke	Consume more asparagus, broccoli, Brussels sprouts, cabbage, cauliflower, spinach, sweet potatoes, turnips, whole grains, nuts, seeds, unpolished brown rice, carrots, pumpkin, squash, yams, apples, berries, Brazil nuts, cantaloupe, cherries, grapes, legumes (including chickpeas, lentils, and red beans), and plums; eat lots of onions and garlic and drink fresh carrot juice daily either alone or mixed with beet juice or asparagus juice; avoid junk foods, processed refined foods, saturated fats, sugar, salt, and white flour products, animal protein (including luncheon meat, hot dogs or smoked or cured meats) except broiled fish (up to 3x/week), avoid

Table 9.4 *(continued)*

Condition	Nutritional Prescription
	peanuts, and limit soybean products); take a multivitamin and multimineral daily and 5,000–20,000 mg vitamin C, 100 mg vitamin B complex, 200 IU (work up to 800 IU gradually) of vitamin E, 25,000[b] IU vitamin A daily
Sinusitis	Test for food sensitivities and avoid foods that test "weak"; drink 6–8 glasses of fluid daily: only water, herb teas, low salt broth or soup; add cayenne and onion to relieve congestion and sinus pressure; increase intake of raw fruits and vegetables to 75% of the diet; drink 10 ounces of fresh carrot juice mixed with 6 ounces of spinach juice daily after noon; take the juice of 1 whole lemon mixed with 4 ounces ground horseradish; drink 1 tablespoon cider vinegar and 1 tablespoon honey in a glass of water at least 3x/day); in addition to a daily multivitamin and multimineral, take: 1,000 to 10,000 mg vitamin C plus bioflavonoids daily in divided doses, 10,000 IU vitamin A daily, and vitamin B complex with at least 100 mg pantothenic acid 3 times a day; avoid mucus-producing foods including cheese, milk, frozen yogurt, whipped cream, and ice cream; avoid sugar, wheat, flours, coffee, alcohol, and salty foods; for an acute infection take: 10,000 mg buffered vitamin C (or whatever amount can be tolerated without developing diarrhea), 200,000 IU vitamin A[b] daily for up to 1 week, then reduce to 25,000 to 50,000 IU (can also use the micelized form, mixed with water as nose drops), 500 to 1,000 mg bee propolis 3x/day; take: acidophilus as per label to replace "good" intestinal bacteria if on antibiotics, quercetin plus bromelain per label to protect against allergens and increase immunity, flaxseed oil as directed on label to reduce pain and inflammation, Pycnogenol or grape seed extract as per label to reduce inflammation and allergic reactions, zinc lozenges every 2–4 waking hours for 1 week to boost immunity
TMJ	Test for food sensitivities; focus on steamed vegetables, fresh fruits, whole grain products, fresh water fish, skinless chicken and turkey, brown rice, and homemade soups and breads; eliminate caffeine, sugar, all white flour products (bread, cereals, pastas, cakes, pies, rolls), candy, colas, potato chips, pies, and fast foods; avoid chewing very large pieces of food or hard brittle food; in addition to a daily multivitamin and multimineral, take: 1,200–2,000 mg calcium chelate or citrate with 600–1,000 mg magnesium in divided doses after meals and at bedtime, 100 mg vitamin B complex with extra pantothenic acid 3x/day
Vaginitis	Test for food sensitivities; eat plain yogurt that contains live cultures or apply yogurt directly to the vagina; eat a diet that is sugar-free, fruit-free, and yeast-free, avoiding aged cheeses, alcohol, chocolate, dried fruits, fermented foods, grain containing gluten (wheat, oats, rye, and barley), ham, honey, nut butters, raw mushrooms, pickles, sprouts, soy

(continued)

Table 9.4 *(continued)*

Condition	Nutritional Prescription
	sauce, sugar in any form, vinegar, and yeast in all forms; during an acute inflammation eliminate citrus and acid fruits (lemons, grapefruits, oranges, pineapples, tomatoes, and limes) totally, then slowly add them back; in addition to a daily multivitamin and multimineral, mineral, take: acido-phyllis as per label to replenish "friendly" bacteria, biotin (inhibits yeast), vitamin B complex as per label (often deficient in individuals with vagini-tis), 1 capsule garlic 3x/day (has antifungal properties), 50,000 IU vitamin A daily[b], and 400 IU vitamin E daily (powerful antioxidants that aid in healing), 2,000–5,000 mg vitamin C daily (necessary for tissue healing)
Varicose Veins	Test for food sensitivities and avoid those that test weak; adopt a high-fiber diet including plenty of fresh fruits, vegetables, and whole grains; daily, after noon, drink 7 ounces fresh carrot juice mixed with 4 ounces celery and 3 ounces spinach juice; at least 2 hours later, drink 10 ounces carrot juice mixed with 3 ounces each beet and cucumber juice; avoid refined foods; in addition to a daily multivitamin and multimineral, take: 400–1,000 mg vitamin E, 1,000 mg bioflavonoids or Pycnogenol daily
Wound Healing (Pre- and Post-Op)	In addition to a daily multivitamin and multimineral, take: powered high potency acidophillus 3x/day (to stabilize intestinal flora), 60 mg coenzyme Q_{10} (to improve tissue oxygenation), 100 mg geranium (oxygenation and pain relief), protein supplement of freeform amino acids to aid healing, 2 garlic capsules 3x/day to enhance immune function, 500 mg L-cystine 2x/day to speed healing, 5,000–10,000 mg vitamin C to aid tissue repair, 400 mg vitamin E daily and apply to wound after stitches have been removed, 80 mg zinc plus 1,500 mg calcium plus 1,000 mg magnesium; eat raw fresh fruits and vegetables; sip filtered water with the juice of a lemon in it throughout the day
Yeast infec-tions	Test for food sensitivities and avoid any that test "weak"; eliminate antibiotics, birth control pills, corticosteroids, and ulcer drugs; begin a yeast- and sugar-free diet including no bread or baked goods with yeast in them; no cheese, mushrooms, vinegar, soy sauce, fermented foods (except unsweetened yogurt), alcohol, cookies, candy, ice cream, diet or regular sodas, dried fruit, chocolate, and sweeteners (sugar, fructose, honey, malt, barley, and juices)

Sources: JF Balch and PA Balch. (1997). *Prescription for Nutritional Healing*. New York, Garden City Park: Avery Publishing; D. Berkson, *The Foot Book*. (1977). New York: Barnes and Noble Books; CC Clark. (1996). *Wellness Practitioner: Concepts, Research, and Strategies*, New York: Springer Publishing Company; R Golan (1995). *Optimal Wellness*. New York: Ballantine Books. JR Lee, J Hanley, & V Hopkins. (1999). *What Your Doctor May Not Tell You About Premenopause*. New York: Warner Books.

[a]Test for acidosis when the following symptoms are present: frequent sighing, insomnia, water retention, recessed eyes, rheumatoid arthritis, migraine headaches, abnormally low blood pressure, dry hard stools, foul-smelling stools accompanied by a burning sensation in the anus, alternating constipation and diarrhea, difficulty swallowing, burning in the mouth and/or under the tongue,

Table 9.4   *(continued)*

sensitivity of the teeth to vinegar and acid fruits and bumps on the roof of the mouth or tongue. If a nitrazine paper test (available at any drugstore) of either saliva or urine tests acid, below pH 7.0, omit acid foods: alcohol, asparagus, beans, Brussels sprouts, chickpeas, cocoa, coffee, cornstarch, eggs, fish, flour products, ketchup, legumes, lentils, meat, milk, mustard, noodles, oatmeal, olives, organ meats, pasta, pepper, plums, poultry, prunes, sauerkraut, shellfish, soft drinks, sugar and all foods with sugar in them, tea and vinegar
[b]Do not exceed 10,000 IU daily if pregnant.
[c]Caution, do not take tyrosine if taking an MAO inhibitor drug.
[d]Avoid if suffering from manic (bipolar) depression.
[e]Do not give to children.

REFERENCES

Balch JF, & Balch PA. (1997). *Prescription for Nutritional Healing.* Garden City Park, NY: Avery Publishing.

Balch JF, & Balch PA. (1990). *Prescription for Nutritional Healing.* Garden City Park, NY: Avery Publishing, pp. 12–13.

Bennett W, & Gurin J. (1982). *The Dieter's Dilemma: Eating Less and Weighing More.* New York: Basic Books.

Davis PA, Gold EG, Hackman RM, Stern JS, & Gershwin ME. (1998). The use of complementary/alternative medicine for the treatment of asthma in the United States. *J Investig Allerg Clin Immunol* 8(2):73–77.

Epstein L, & Weng R. (1980). Aerobic exercise and weight. *Additive Behaviors* 5:371–388.

Gwinup G. (1975). Effect of exercise alone on the weight of obese females. *Arch Int Med* 135:676–680.

Lappe F. (1975). *Diet for a small plant.* New York: Ballantine, pp. 62–117.

Miller WC, Niederpruem MG, Wallace JP, & Lindeman AK. (1994). Dietary fat, sugar, and fiber predict fat content. *J of the Am Diet Assoc* 94(6):612–615.

Phinney S, et al. (1980). Capacity for moderate exercise in obese subjects after adaptation to a hypocaloric ketogenic diet. *J Clin Investig* 66:1152–1161.

Simpson H, et al. (1981). A high carbohydrate leguminous diet improves all aspects of diabetic control. *Lancet* 7(8210):1–5.

Skobak-Kaczynski J, & Andersen L. (1975). The effect of a high-level of habitual physical activity in the regulation of fatness during aging. *Internatl Arch Occupt & Environm. Hlth.* 36:41–46.

10

HERBS

Plants have been used as treatments since before recorded history. Physical evidence of herbal remedies was found in the 60,000-year old burial site of a Neanderthal man. Herbalists believed that the healing energy inherent in living plants may account for some of their power. This theory is currently being explored by contemporary practitioners (Somerville, 1997).

At one time in the West, herbs were well-researched. Numerous studies were published as late as the mid 20th century. With the advent of synthetic medicines, research was discontinued (Mowry, 1986). Now, the pendulum is swinging back to a science of health as a holistic, rather than a "magic bullet" approach. Herbs are part of that holistic approach. Current interest in herbs also follows on the heels of the realization that medicinal drugs are more expensive, cause many more side effects or allergic reactions, and may not provide adequate treatment for many conditions. For example, aspirin and acetaminophen may actually increase the transmission of cold viruses and extend the duration of a cold (Graham et al., 1990).

HERBAL EFFECTIVENESS

Herbal effectiveness is influenced by the following: (1) growing conditions (soil, insect control and fertilization), (2) climactic conditions (temperature and rainfall), (3) harvesting procedures (when and how the herb is harvested), (4) curing procedures, (5) processing and preparation methods, (6) packaging, (7) storage, and (8) shelf life (Mowry, 1990).

Most of these variables can be controlled if the final product is standardized. This is not an easy process because it is difficult to pin down biological activity to one, or at least a few, constituents. Numerous difficulties and pitfalls can occur. It is necessary to identify which herbs will benefit from extraction and standardization, which are more effective in their natural state, and which will lose potency when made more bio-available.

United States research in standardization of herbs is in its infancy. Herbal investigations in Germany, Italy, Russia, Switzerland, and France have begun to identify active herbal constitutents and standardize them for purchase. Guaranteed Potency Herbs can begin to answer the complaint that the active material in any given batch is suspect. Guaranteed Potency Herbs are guaranteed by the manufacturer to contain the advertised amount of the active ingredient (Mowry, 1990). If practitioners do recommend herbs, it makes sense to suggest clients use guaranteed potency herbs.

HERBS AND THEIR EFFECTS

Table 10.1 provides information on herbs that have stood the test of animal, laboratory, and/or human studies and have proven their effectiveness over time (Mowry, 1990).

Table 10.1   Herbs and Their Effects*

Herb	Effect	Toxicity
Aloe Vera	Enhancing survival in individuals with advanced solid tumors (Lissoni, et al., 1998); enhances dermal wound healing (Chithra et al., 1998a; Heggers, et al., 1997) and diabetic wound healing (Chithra et al., 1998b); may reduce symptoms of and for children fibromyalgia chronic fatigue (Dykman et al., 1998); prevents UVB-induced accessory cell function due to radiation (Lee et al., 1997); acts as an immunostimulant (Stuart et al., 1997); has antiinflammatory action (Vazquez, 1996); treats psoriasis (Syed et al., 1996); laxative, up to 30 ml/dose; antiseptic and anti-hepatitis (Wirth, 1998)	Commercially prepared aloe vera gels may contain added toxins (Avila et al., 1997); by mouth doses contraindicated during pregnancy and for children

(continued)

Table 10.1   *(continued)*

Herb	Effect	Toxicity
Artichoke	Acts as an antioxidant (Brown & Rice-Evans, 1998; Gebhardt, 1997); inhibits cholesterol bysnthesis (Gebhardt, 1998); provides anticancer activity (Mukhtar & Agarwal, 1996; Yasukawa et al., 1996)	Not toxic
Bilberry	Protects the heart against prolonged stress exposure (Marcollet et al., 1970); possesses good anti-inflammatory (Bonacina et al., 1973) and antiviral activity (Fokina et al., 1991); provides anticancer activity (Bomser et al., 1996); inhibits cholesterol-induced atherosclerosis (Kadar et al., 1979); possesses anti-thrombotic activity (Gomez-Serranillos et al., 1983); treats severe myopia (Barradah, 1967); treats retinal disturbances and chronic visual fatigue (Chevaleraud & Perdriel, 1968); reduces blood purpuras, varicose veins, and various central nervous system circulation problems (Terrasse & Moinade, 1964); treats phlebitis to hypertension, including fragility associated with diabetes, in conditions involving breakdown of capillary walls (Thomas & Barisain, 1965; Sevin, 1966; Coget & Merlin, 1968; Guermonprez & Miltgen, 1972/1973); stimulates peripheral circulation (Terrasse et al., 1969); reduces disorders of blood ves-	Not toxic

Table 10.1 *(continued)*

Herb	Effect	Toxicity
	sels in the conjunctiva of diabetic and prediabetic clients with tendencies toward glaucoma (Romani, 1969); provides antispasmodic and central nervous system sedative action (Canivet & Passa, 1971); anti-diarrheal, vs. edema, vs. pharyngitis (Wirth, 1998)	
Black Cohosh	Treats symptoms of menopause (Lieberman, 1998)	Overdoses or long-term use can lead to dizziness, diarrhea, nausea, vomiting, abdominal pain, joint pains, headaches, and lowered heart rate, liver problems, breast tumors, abnormal clotting; not to be used when pregnant
Butcher's Broom (ruscus aculeatus whole herb only)	Treats hemorrhoids (Lemozy et al., 1976; Pris, 1977); improves circulation disorders of the legs (Cohen, 1977; Sterboul, 1962); phlebitis (Capra, 1972); anti-inflammatory (Wirth, 1998)	Occasional nausea or gastritis
Capsaicin (Hot red pepper)	Antioxidant and anti-inflammatory (Surh et al., 1998); decreases pain of shingles and other pains (Wirth, 1998); anticarcinogen (Wirth, 1998)	Not toxic
Centella	Treats arteriosclerosis (Hachen & Bourgoin, 1979); accelerates skin healing (Faris, 1960; Fincato, 1960; Maleville, 1979); reduces lesions and ulcerative problems associated with pregnancy (Remotti & Colombo, 1962; Baudon-Gladdier, 1963; Heller, 1968); healing after tonsilectomy (Pignataro & Teatini, 1965); counteracts negative effects of	Not toxic

(continued)

Table 10.1   *(continued)*

Herb	Effect	Toxicity
	radiotherapy after surgery (Colonna d'Istria & Savy, 1970); treats venous insufficiency including varices and phlebitis (Allegra, 1984; Mazolla & Gini, 1982); reduces heaviness of the legs, tingling, and nocturnal cramps (Boely, 1975); treats cellulitis, including erysipelas (Bailly, 1976; Cezes & Combalie, 1976)	
Chamomile	Anti-inflammatory and immunoregulator for rheumatoid arthritis and lymphomas (You et al., 1998); relaxes digestive and nervous systems	Not toxic except for anyone allergic to plants in the daisy family
Curcumin/ Turmeric	Enhances wound healing (Sidhu et al., 1998); anti-inflammatory, anti-mutagenic and chemo-prevention agent (Jaruga et al., 1998; Huang et al., 1998; Ranjan et al., 1998; Gautam et al., 1998); protects the kidney (Shoskes, 1998); vs. arthritis and scabies (Wirth, 1998)	Not toxic
Echinacea	Prevents and treats various bacterial and viral infections (Koch & Uebel, 1953; Koch & Uebel, 1954); activates macrophages and possibly T-cells that destroy cancerous cells and foreign intracellular invaders (Wacker & Hilbig, 1978); anti-inflammatory (Tragini et al., 1985); vs. recurrent candidal vaginitis, URIs, radiation, leukemia, colon	Not toxic, but should be taken a few weeks on and a few off through the year

Table 10.1 *(continued)*

Herb	Effect	Toxicity
	CA (Wirth, 1998); reduces incidence and severity of cold symptoms (Braunig, 1993; Schoneberger, 1992)	
Garlic	Treats hepatopulmonary (Abrahams & Fallon, 1998); anti-tumor effect (Chen et al., 1998); reduces clotting activity (Bordia et al., 1998); reduces blood fats and blood pressure (Steiner & Lin, 1998); antimicrobial (Yoshida et al., 1998); antifungal (Wirth, 1998)	Not toxic
Ginger	Anti-emetic that reverses GI effects of cancer therapy (Sharma & Gupta, 1988); antioxidative and anti-inflammatory (Park et al., 1998); lowers cholesterol (Bhandari et al., 1998); anti-tumor activity (Surh et al., 1998); reduces post-operative nausea (Visalyaputra et al., 1998); prevents aflatoxin-related cancer (Wirth, 1998)	Not toxic; Heartburn in some individuals
Ginkgo Biloba	Improves blood brain flow and memory (Haan et al., 1982; Rai et al., 1991); improves ringing in the ears and vertigo (Gaby, 1996); cognitive activator that treats Alzheimer's (Itil et al., 1998; Kanowski et al., 1996); and dementia (LeBars, 1997); vs. intermittent claudication (Wirth, 1998); vs. PMS-related breast engorgement (Wirth, 1998); vs. vertigo (Wirth, 1998)	Not toxic; Occasional reports of GI upset, headache or rash (Somerville, 1997)

(continued)

Table 10.1   *(continued)*

Herb	Effect	Toxicity
American Ginseng	Anti-stress, antipsychotic, antipyretic, hypotensive, anticonvulsant, analgesic, tranquilizer (Takagi, 1973; Kim et al., 1971); vs. stress induced GI ulcer (Wirth, 1998); vs. post op stress (Wirth, 1998)	Not toxic; Asthmatics may experience an attack; palpitations, increased blood pressure or postmenopausal bleeding have been reported (Somerville, 1997)
Panax Ginseng	Activates brain activity; hypertensive, antifatigue; enhances intellectual performance, stimulates DNA synthesis (Takagi et al., 1973; Wang et al., 1983; Han et al., 1998)	Not toxic (See American Ginseng)
Goldenseal	Vs. Diarrhea, tumors, hepatic toxins (Wirth, 1998)	Contraindicated during pregnancy; Moderate doses may increase cardiac output and peripheral vasoconstriction; More than 500 mg/day may cause CNS toxicity
Gota Kola	Vs. bladder lesions, cancer; apply topically for psoriasis and wound healing (Wirth, 1998)	Safe; Handling leaves can cause dermatitis
Green onion	Antifungal (Yin & Cheng, 1998) for A. flavus even at 80 degrees C.	Not toxic
Green tea	Vs. cancer (Agarwal & Mukhtar, 1996)	May increase glucose and blood pressure
Hawthorne berry	Dilates coronary arteries; decreases peripheral vascular resistance; vs. angina (Wirth, 1998)	Hypotension; arrthymias (Wirth, 1998)
Kava-Kava	Oral anesthetic; Sedative (Wirth, 1998); reduces anxiety (Kinzler, Kromer & Lehmann, 1991)	Dermatitis; hematuria, weakness, decreased WBC, pulmonary hypertension possible if more than 1 cup TID taken (Wirth, 1998)
Licorice	Antibacterial action (Haraguchi et al., 1998); antioxidant action (Belinky et al., 1998)	Avoid if pregnant; Large amounts can raise blood pressure and lead to edema and loss of potassium (Wirth, 1998)

Table 10.1 *(continued)*

Herb	Effect	Toxicity
Milk Thistle	Treats mushroom poisoning (Vogel, 1980; Floersheim, et al., 1982); attenuates nitrus oxide that is correlated with neurodegenerative diseases (Soliman & Mazzio, 1998); provides anticarcinogenic effects (Zi & Feyes, 1998; Katiyar et al., 1997); prevents atherosclerotic changes (Bialecka, 1997); treats liver disease (Flora et al., 1998; Dehmlow et al., 1996; Ferenci et al., 1989);protects kidney (von Schonfeld et al., 1997); may treat noninsulin-dependent diabetes mellitus (von Schonfeld et al., 1997); inhibits cyclic AMP breakdown (Koch et al., 1985)	Not toxic; loose stools may occur due to increased bile secretion (Somerville, 1997)
Motherwort	Suppresses mammary tumors (Nagasawa et al., 1992); induces resistance to viral infection (Fokina et al., 1991); reduces blood hyperviscosity (Zou et al., 1989)	
Mullein	Vs. pharyngitis (Wirth, 1998)	Not toxic (Wirth, 1998)
Oregano	Bactericidal activity (Ultee et al., 1998)	Not toxic
Pennyroyal	None	Severe or fatal effects may occur; stimulates abortion (Wirth, 1998)
Peppermint	Vs. irritable bowel syndrome; relaxant, stimulates bile (Wirth, 1998)	May worsen hiatal hernia or gastro-esophageal reflex disease (Wirth, 1998)
Rosemary	May lower total cholesterol (Lopez-Bote et al., 1998)	Not toxic
Sage	May lower total cholesterol (Lopez-Bote et al., 1998);	Not toxic but avoid if epileptic hypertensive or pregnant (Wirth, 1998)

(continued)

Table 10.1 *(continued)*

Herb	Effect	Toxicity
	antimicrobial, antioxidant and antispasmodic (Wirth, 1998)	
Saw Palmetto	Treats benign prostatic hyperplasia (Gerber et al., 1998); vs. allergies; anti-inflammatory (Wirth, 1998)	Not toxic; Avoid if pregnant; more than 300 mg/day may aggravate estrogen-sensitive tumors (Wirth, 1998)
Schizandra	Improves learning (Nishiyama et al., 1996); Treats liver cancer (Ohtaki et al., 1996); powerful antioxidant (Zhao et al., 1990)	Potential drug interactions; CNS depression, mutagenicity (Wirth, 1998)
St. John's Wort	Reduces depression (Nordfors & Harvig, 1997; Linde et al., 1996)	High blood pressure, headaches, nausea, and vomiting, and photosensitivity; possible drug interactions as for MAO inhibitors
Thyme	Bactericidal activity (Ultee et al., 1998); insecticial action (Morsy et al., 1998)	Not toxic
Valerian	Treats sleep disorders (Schmitz & Jackel, 1998)	Safe; no hangover effects the following morning (Schmitz & Jackel, 1998)

*Use standardized herbs as suggested on the bottle; consult a herb book (e.g., Keville or Mowry for dosages and use).

COMBINING HERBAL SUPPLEMENTS WITH PRESCRIPTION DRUGS

Although herbalists do not advise combining prescription drugs with herbs, there are ways to combine them, but the following steps are suggested when doing so:

1. Read package inserts of any prescription drugs clients are currently taking.
2. Ensure there is no caution against taking any herbs or other substance together with the prescription drug(s).
3. Be familiar with related research. Suggest the type and dosage used to produce research results, if possible.

4. Contact the Office of Alternative Medicine Clearinghouse, (888)644-6226, or visit its Web site at http://altmed.od.nih.gov. OAM provides an exchange of information between complementary practitioners. Fact sheets are available on some herbal products.
5. Consult with a community herbalist you trust. (This presupposes networking with complementary therapists and knowing their strengths and weaknesses.)
6. If no community herbalist is available, call the Herb Research Foundation (303-449-2265) or visit their web site: www.herbs.org, for information on specific herbs.

REFERENCES

Abrahams GA, & Fallon MB. (1998). Treatment of hepatopulmonary syndrome with Allium sativum L. (garlic): a pilot trial. *J Clin Gastroenterol* 27(3):232–235.

Agarwal R, & Mukhtar H. (1996). Cancer chemoprevention by polyphenols in green tea and artichokes. *Adv Exp Med Biol* 401:35–50.

Allegra C. (1984). Studio capillaroscopico comparativo tra alcuni bioflavonoidi e frazione totale triterpenica di centella asiatica nell insufficienza venosa. *Clin Terr* 110:555.

Avila B, Rivero J, Herrera F, & Fraile G. (1997). Cytotoxicity of a low molecular weight fraction from Aloe vera (Aloe barbadensis Miller) gel. *Toxicon* 35(9):1423–1430.

Bailly PJ. (1976). Une nouvelle therapeutique de la cellulite par l'extrait de centella asiatica. *Med Prat* 629:37.

Barradah M, Shourkey I, & Hegazy M. (1967). Difarel 100 in the treatment of retinal vascular disorders and high myopia. *Bull Opthal. Soc. Egypt* 60:251.

Baudon-Gladdier B. (1963). Lesion perineals et asiaticoside. *Gaz Med France* 70:2463.

Belinky PA, Aviram M, Mahmood S, & Vaya J. (1998). Structural aspects of the inhibitory effect of glabridin on LDL oxidation. *Free Radic Biol Med* 24(9):1419–1429.

Bhandari U, Sharma JN, & Zafar R. (1998). The protective action of ethanolic ginger (Zingiber officinale) extract in cholesterol fed rabbits. *J Ethnopharmacol* 61(2):167–171.

Bialecka M. (1997). The effect of bioflavonoids (milk thistle) and lecithin on the course of experimental atherosclerosis in rabbits. *Ann Acad Med Stetin* 43:41–56.

Boely C. (1975). Indications therapeutiques de l'extrait titre de centella asiatica en phlebologie. *Gaz Med France* 82:741.

Bomser J, Madhavi DL, Singletary K, & Smith MA. (1996). In vitro anticancer activity of fruit extracts from Vaccinium species. *Planta Med* 62(3):212–216.

Bonacina F, Galliani G, & Pacciano F. (1973). Attivita degli antocianosidi nei processi flogistici acuti. *Famaceo* ed. pr. 28:428.

Bordia A, Verma SK, & Srivastave KC. (1998). Effect of garlic (Allium satiuum) on blood lipids, blood sugar, fibrinogen, & fibrinolytic activity in patients with coronary artery disease. *Essent Fatty Acids* 58(4):257–263.

Braunig, B. (1993). Echinacea purpurea radix for strengthening immune response in flu-like infections. *Z. Phytother* 13:7–13.

Brown JE, & Rice-Evans CA. (1998). Luteolin-rich artichoke extract protects low density lipoprotein from oxidation in in vitro. *Free Radical Res* 29(3):247–255.

Burger RA, Torres AP, Waram RP, Caldwell VD, & Hughes BG. (1997). Echinacea-induced cytokine production by human macrophages. *Int J. Immunopharmacol* 19(7):371–379.

Cahn J, Herold M, & Senault B. (1964). Antiphlogistic and anti-inflammatory activity of F 191. Int. Symp Non-Steroidal Anti-inflammatory Drugs. Milano, Italy.

Canivet J, & Passa Ph. (1971). Interet therapeutique d'une association d'anthocyanosides, d'antispasmodiques et de neuro-sedatif central. *G.M. de France* 78:682.

Capra C. (1972). Studio farmacologico e tossicologico di componenti del ruscus aculeatus L. *Fitoterapia* 43:99.

Cezes A, & Combalie JC. (1976). 477 cas de cellulite traites par madecassol. *J Med Esthetique* 3(12):31.

Chen DW, Ching JG, Hsieh CL, & Lin JG. (1998). Effects of garlic components diallyl sulfide and di allyl disulfide on arylamine *N*-acetyltransferase activity in human colon tumour cells. *Food Chem Toxicol* 36(9–10):761–770.

Chevaleraud J, & Perdriel G. (1968). Peut-on ameliorer la vision nocturne des aviateurs. *Gaz Med de France* 18:25.

Chevillard L, Ranson M, & Senault B. (1964). Activite anti-iflammatoire d'extraits de fragon epineux (ruscus aculeatus L.). *Med Pharmacol Exp* 12:109–114.

Chithra P, Sajithal GB, & Chandrakasan G. (1998a). Influence of Aloe vera on collagen characteristics in healing dermal wounds in rats. *Mol Cell Biochem* 181(1–2):71–76.

Chithra P, Sajithal GB, & Chandrakasan G. (1998b). Influence of aloe vera on the healing of dermal wounds in diabetic rats. *J Ethnopharmacol* 59(3):195–201.

Coget J, & Merlen (1968). Etude clinique d'un nouvel agent de protection vasculaire, le Difrarel 20, composed' anthocyanosides isoles de v. myrtillus. *Phlebolgie* 2:221.

Cohen J. (1977). Fraitement par le ruscus des incidences veineuses de la contraception orald. *Vie Medicale* 10:1305.

Colonna d'lstria J, & Savy P. (1970). Recherche sur l'action cicatrisante du madecassol en chirugie cervicale et laryngee, apres radiations. *JFORL* 19:507.

de la Motte S, Bose-O'Reilly S, Heinisch M, & Harrison F. (1997). Double-blind comparison of an apple pectin-chamomile extract preparation with placebo in children with diarrhea. *Arzneimittelforschung* 47(11):1247–1249.

Dehmlow C, Erhard J, & de Groot H. (1996). Inhibition of Kupffer cell functions as an explanation for the hepatoprotective properties of silibinin. *Hepatology* 23(4):749–754.

Dykman KD, Tone C, Ford C, & Dykman RA. (1998). The effects of nutritional supplements on the symptoms of fibromyalgia and chronic fatigue syndrome. *Integr Physiol Behav Sci* 33(1):61–71.

Facino RM, Carini M, Stefain R, Aldini G, & Saibene B. (1995). Anti-elastase and anti-hyaluronidase activities of saponins and sapogenins from Herdera helix, Aesculus hippocastanum and Ruscus aculeatus: Factors contributing to their efficacy in the treatment of venous insufficiency. *Arch Pharm (Weinheim)* 328(10):720–724.

Faris G. (1960). L'azione terapeutica dell'asiaticoside in campo dermatological. *Minerva Med* 51:2244.

Ferenci P, Dragosics B, Dittrich H, Frank H, Brenda L, Lochs H, Meryn S, Base W, & Schneider B. (1989). Randomized controlled trial of Silyman treatment in patients with cirrhosis of the liver. *J Hepatol* 9(1):105–113.

Fincato M. (1960). Sul trattamento di lesioni cutanee con estratto di'centella asiatica. *Minerva Med* 15:1235.

Floersheim GL, Weber O, Tschumi P, & Ulbrich M. (1982). Die klinishche knollenblaetter-pilzvergiftung (amanita phalloides): prognotishce faktoren und therapeutishche massnahmen. (Eine analyse analyse anhand von 205 faellen.) Schweiz. *Medizinische WochenAschrift* 112:1164–1177.

Flora K, Hahn M, Rosen H, & Renner K. (1998). Milk thistle Silybum marianum) for the therapy of liver disease. *Am J. Gastroenterol* 93(2):139–143.

Fokina GI, Frolova TV, Toikleh' VM, & Pogodina VV. (1991). Experimental phytotherapy of tick-borne encephalitis. *Vopr Virusol* 36(1):18–21.

Gaby AR. (1996). Ginkgo biloba extract: A review. *Alt Med Rev* 1(4):236–242.

Gautam SC, Xu YX, Pindolia KR, Janakiraman N, & Chapman RA. (1998). Nonselective inhibition of proliferation of transformed and nontransformed cells by the anticancer agent curcumin (diferulcylmethane). *Biochem Pharmacol* 55(8):1333–1337.

Gebhardt R. (1997). Antioxidative and protective properties of extracts from leaves of the artichoke (Cynara scolymus L.) against hydroperoxide-induced oxidative stress in cultured rat hepatocytes. *Toxicol Appl Pharmacol* 144(2):279–286.

Gebhardt R. (1998). Inhibition of cholesterol bisynthesis in primary cultured rat hepatocytes by artichoke (Cynara scolymus L.) extracts. *J Pharmacol Exp Ther* 286(3):1122–1128.

Gerber GS, Zagaja GP, Bales GT, Chodak GW, & Contreras, BA. (1998). Saw palmetto (Serenoa repens) in men with lower urinary tract symptoms: Effects of urodynamic parameters and voiding symptoms. *Urology* 51(6):1003–1007.

Gomez-Serranillos FM, Zaragoza F, & Alvarez P. (1983). efectos sobre la agegacion plaquetaria in vitro de los antocianosidos del vaccinium mytrillus L. *An R. Acad Farm* 49:79.

Graham NM, Burell CJ, Douglas RM, Debelle P, & Davies L. (1990). Adverse effects of aspirin, acetaminophen, and ibruprofen on immune function, viral shredding and clinical status in rhinovirus-infested volunteers. *J Infect Dis* 162(6):1277–1282.

Guermonprez JL, & Miltgen M. (1972–1973). Action des anthocyanosides de vaccinium myrtillus sure la resistance capilaire chez l'hypertendu et la diabetique (a propos de 40 observations). *Vie Med* 21:6.

Hachen A, & Bourgoin JY. (1979). Etude anatomo-clinique des effect de l'extrait titre de centella asiatica dans la lipodystrophie localisee. *Med Prat* 738 (Supplement):7.

Haan J, Reekermann V, Welter FL, Sabin G, & Muller E. (1982) Ginkgo biloba flavongly-koside. Therapiemoglichkeit der zerebralen insuffizienz. *Medizinische Welt* 33:1001.

Haraguchi H, Tanimoto K, Tamura Y, Mizutani K, & Kinoshita I. (1998). Mode of antibacterial action of retrochalcones from Glycyrrhiza inflata. *Phytochemistry* 48(1):125–129.

Huang MT, Lou YR, Xie JG, Ma W, Lu YP, Yen P, Zhu BT, Newmark H, & Ho CT. (1998). Effect of dietary curcumin and dibenzoyimethane on formation of 7,12-dimethylbenzialanthra-cene-induced mammary tumors and lymphomas/leukemias in Sencar mice. *Carcinogenesis* 19(91):1697–1700.

Han KH, Choe SC, Kim HS, Sohn DW, Nam KY, Oh BH, Lee MM, Park YB, Choi YS, Seo JD, & Lee YW. (1998). Effect of red ginseng on blood pressure in patients with essential hypertension and white coat hypertension. *Am J Clin Med* 26(21):199–209.

Heggers JP, Elzaim H, Garfield R, Goodheart R, Listengarten D, Zhao J, & Phillips LG. (1997). *J Altern Complem Med* 3(2):149–153.

Heller L. (1968) Madecassol en gynecologie. *Gaz Med France* 32:6626.

Itil T, & Martorano D. (1998). Natural substances in psychiatry (Gingko biloba in dementia). *Psychopharm. Bull* 31(1):147–158.

Jaruga E, Bielak-Zmijewska A, Sikora E, Skierski J, Radziszewska E, Piwooka K, & Bartosz G. (1998). Glutathione-independent mechanism of apoptosis inhibition by curcumin in rat thymocytes. *Biochem Pharmacol* 56(8):961–965.

Kadar A, Robert L, Miskulin M, Tixier JM, Breachemier D, & Robert AM. (1979). Influence of anthocyanoside treatment on the cholesterol-induced atherosclerosis in the rabbit. *Paroi Arter* 5:181.

Kanowski S, Herrmann WM, Stephan K, Wierich W, & Horr R. (1996) Proof of efficacy of the Ginkgo biloba special extract EGb 761 in outpatients suffering from ild to moderate primary degenerative dementia of the Alzheimer type or multi-infarct dementia. *Pharmacopsychiatry* 29(2):47–56.

Katiyar SK, Korman NJ, Mukhtar H, & Agarwal R. (1997). Protective effects of silymarin against photocarcinogenesis in a mouse skin model. *J Natl Cancer Inst* 89(8):556–566.

Kazaki T, Monsaki N, Shiina R, & Sato Y. (1998). Role of transforming growth factor-beta pathway in the mechanism of wound healing by saponin from Ginseng Radix ruba. *Br J Pharmacol* 125(2):255–262.

Keville K. (1996). *Herbs for Health and Healing.* Emmaus, PA: Rodale Press, Inc.

Kim EC, Cho HY, & Kim JM. (1971). Effect of panax ginseng on the central nervous system. *Korean J. Pharmacol* 2:23–28.

Kinzler E, Kromer J, & Lehman. (1991). Clinical efficacy of a kova extract in patients with anxiety syndrome: Double-blind placebo controlled study over 4 weeks. *Arzneimittel-Forsch* 41:584–588.

Koch E, & Uebel H. (1953). Experimental studies concerning the local action of echinacea purpurea on tissues. *Arzneimittel-Forschung* 3:16–19.

Koch E, & Uebel H. (1954). Experimental studies on the local influence of cortisone and echinacin upon tissue resistance against streptococcus infection. *Arzneimittel-Forschung* 4:424–426.

Koch HP, Bachner J, & Loffler E. (1985). Silymarin: potent inhibitor of cyclic AMP phosphodiesterase. *Methods Find Exp Clin Pharmacol* 7(8):409–413.

LeBars PL, Katz MM, & Berman N. (1997). A placebo-controlled, double-blind, randomized trial of an extract of *Ginkgo biloba* for dementia. *J Amer Med Assoc* 2778(16):1327–1332.

Lee CK, Han SS, Mo YK, Kim RS, Chung MH, Park YI, Lee SK, & Kim YS. (1997). Prevention of ultraviolet radiation suppression of accessory cell function of Langerhans cells by Aloe vera gel components. *Immunopharmacology* 37(2):153–162.

Lemozy J, Suduce P, Garrigues JM, & Saint-Pieer A. (1976). Interet du proctolog dans le traitment des hemorroides et des fissures anales. *Mediterranee Med* 92:87.

Lieberman S. (1998). A review of the effectiveness of Cimicifriga racemosa (black cohosh) for the symptoms of menopause. *J Women's Health* 7(5): 525–529.

Linde K, Ramirez G, Mulrow CD, Pauls A, Weidenhammer W, & Melchart D. St. John's Wort for depression—an overview and meta-analysis of randomised clinical trials. *Brit Med J* 313(7052):253–258.

Lissoni P, Giani L, Zerbini S, Trabattoni P, & Ravelli F. (1998). Biotherapy with the Pineal Immunomodulating Hormone Melatonin versus Melatonin plus Aloe vera in untreatable advanced solid neoplasms. *Nat Immun* 16(1):27–33.

Lopez-Bote CJ, Gray JI, Gomaai EA, & Flegal CJ. (1998). Effect of dietary administration of oil extracts from rosemary and sage on lipid oxidation in broiler meat. *Br Poult Sci* 39(2):235–240.

Maleville J. (1979). Etude clinicque d'un nouveau tulle gras. *Gaz Med Ital* 86:593.

Marcollet M, Bastide P, & Tronche P. (1970). Effet angio-protecteur des anthocyanosides de vaccinium myrtillus objective vis-a-vis de la liberation de la lactate dehydrogenase (LDH) et de ses isoenzymers cardiaques chez le rat soumis a une epreuve de nage. *C.R. Soc Biol* 183:1786.

Mazzola M, & Gini MM. (1982). La centella asiatica nella terapia della insufficienza venos cronica. Ricerca clinica controllata a cecita doppia vs placebo. *Clin Europ* 21:160.

McKenna J. (1998). *Natural Alternatives to Antibiotics*. Garden City Park, NY: Avery Publishing Group.

Melchart D, Linde K, Worku F, Sarkady S, Holzman M, Jurcic K, & Wagner H. (1995). Results of 5 randomized studies on the immunodulatory activity of preparations of Echinacea. *J Altern Comple Med* 1(2):145–160.

Morsy TA, Shoukry A, Mazyad SA, & Makled KM. (1998). *J Egypt Soc Parasitol* 28(2):503–510.

Mowry D. (1986). *The Scientific Validation of Herbal Medicine*. New Canaan, CT: Keats Publishing, Inc.

Mowry D. (1990). *Next Generation Herbal Medicine*. New Canaan, CT: Keats Publishing, Inc.

Mowry D. (1993). *Herbal Tonic Therapies*. New Canaan, CT: Keats Publishing, Inc.

Mukhtar H, & Agarwal R. (1996). Skin cancer chemoprevention. *J Investig Dermatol Symp Proc* 1(2):209–214.

Nagasawa H, Inatomi H, Suzuki M, & Mori T. (1992). Further study on the effects of motherwort (Leonurus sibiricus L) on preneoplastic and neoplastic mammary gland growth in multiparous GR/A mice. *Anticancer Res* 12(1):141–143.

Nishiyama N, Chu PJ, & Saito H. (1996). An herbal prescription S-113m consisting of biota, ginseng and schizandra, improves learning performance in senescence accelerated mouse. *Biol Pharm Bull* 19(3):388–393.

Nordfors M, & Hartvig, P. (1997). St. John's Wort against depression. *Lakartidningen* 94(25):2365–2367.

Ohtaki Y, Hida T, Hiramatsu K, Kanitani M, Ohshima T, Nomura M, & Miyamoto II. (1996). Deoxycholic acid as an endogenous risk factor for hepatocarcinogenesis and effects of gomisin A, a lignan component of Schizandra fruits. *Anticancer Res* 16(2):751–755.

Park KK, Chun KS, Lee JM, Lee SS, & Surh YJ. (1998). Inhibitory effects of (6)-gingerol, a major pungent principle of ginger, on phorbol ester-induced inflammation, epidermal ornithine decarboxylast activity and skin tumor promotion in ICR mice. *Cancer Lett* 129(2):139–144.

Peters H, Kieser M, & Holscher U. (1998). The efficacy of gingko biloba special extract Egb 761 on intermittent claudication-a placebo controlled double blind multicenter trial. *Vasa* 27(2):106–110.

Pidoux B. (1986). Effects of ginkgo biloba extract on functional activity of the brain. *Presse Med* 15(31):1588–1591.

Pignataro O, & Teatini GP. (1965). Ricera clinica sull'azione cicatrizzante del madecassol nei confronti della mucosa orofaringea. *Minera Med* 56:2683.

Pris J. (1977). Proctolog: Utilisation dans un service d'hematologie. *Gaz Med France* 84:2423.

Rai GS, Shovlin C, & Wesnes KA. (1991). A double-blind placebo-controlled study of ginkgo biloba extract in elderly outpatients with mild to moderate memory impairment. *Curr Med Res Opin* 12(6):350–355.

Ranjan D, Johnston TD, Wu G, Elliott L, Bondad S, & Nagabhushan M. (1998). Curcumin blocks cyclosporine A-resistant CD28 costimulatory pathway of human T-cell proliferation. *J Surg Res* 77(2):174–178.

Romani JD. (1969). Action des anthocyanosides sur l'angiopathie conjonctivale au cours du diabete et du prediabete. *Vie Medicale*, Dic.

Schoneberger D. (1992). The influence of immune-stimulating effects of pressed juice from echinacea purpurea on the course and severity of colds. *Forum Immunologie* 8:2–12.

Schmitz M, & Jackel M. (1998). Randomized, double-blind, controlled clinical trial in parallel group design of hop-valerian preparation compared with a benzodiazepine preparation in patients suffering from sleep disorders. *Wien Med Wochenschr* 148(13):291–293.

Sevin R, & Cuendet JF. (1966). Effets d'une association d'anthocyanosides demyrtille et de beto-carotene sur la resistance capillaire des diabetiques. *Opthalmologica* 152:109.

Sharma SS, & Gupta YK. (1998). Reversal of cisplatin-induced delay in gastric emptying in rats by ginger. *J Ethnopharmacol* 62(1):49–55.

Shoskes DA. (1998). Effect of bioflavonoids quercetin and curcumin on ischemic renal injury: A new class of reno-protective agents. *Transplantation* 66(2):147–152.

Sidhu GS, Singh AK, Thaloor D, Banaudha KK, Patnalk GK, Srimal RC, & Maheshwari RK. (1998). Enhancement of sound healing by curcumin in animals. *Wound Repair Regen* 6(2):167–177.

Soliman KF, & Mazzio EA. (1998). In vitro attenuation of nitric oxide product in C6 astrocyte cell culture by various dietary compounds. *Proc Soc Exp Biol Med* 218(4):390–397.

Somerville R. (1997). *Herbal therapies.* The Alternative Advisor. New York: Time Life Inc.

Steiner M, & Lin RS. (1998). Changes in platelet function and susceptibility of lipoproteins to oxidation associated with administration of aged garlic extract. *J Cardiovasc Pharmocol* 31(6):904–908.

Sterboul K. (1962). Etude clinique d'un vasomoteur veineux. Extrait de fragon epineux. *Gaz Hop Cilils et Militaires* 134:375.

Stuart RW, Lefkowitz DL, Lincoln JA, Howard K, Gelderman, MP, & Lefkowitz SS. (1997). Upregulation of phagocytosis and candidicidal activity of macrophages exposed to the immuno-stimulant accemannan. *Int J Immunopharmacol* 19(2):75–82.

Surh YJ, Lee W, & Lee JM. (1998). Chemoprotective properties of some pungent ingredients present in red pepper and ginger. *Mutat Res* 402(1-2):259–267.

Syed TA, Ahmad SA, Holt AH, Ahmad SA, Ahmad SH, & Afzal M. (1996). Management of psoriasis with Aloe vera extract in a hydrophilic cream: A placebo-controlled, double-blind study. *Trop Med Int Health* 1(4):505–509.

Takagi K. (1973). Pharmacological studies of some oriental medicinals. *Yakhak Hoeji* 17(1):1–8.

Terrasse J, & Moinade S. (1964). Premiers resultats obtenus avec un nouveau facteur vitaminique P'Les anthocyanosides'extraits du v. myrtillus. *Presse Med* 72:397.

Terrasse J, Aubiet-Cuvelier JL, & Marcheix JC. (1969). Action des anthocyanocides sur la circulation perpherique et le test de Landis. *Vie Medicale*, Dic.

Thomas CH, & Barisain P. (1965). L'action des anthocyanosides sur al fagilite des capillaires oculaire dans le diabete et l'hypertension arterielle. *Bull Soc Ophtalm Fran* 65:212.

Thompson KD. (1998). Antiviral activity of Viracea (echinachea and benzalkonium chloride) against acyclovir susceptible and resistant strains of herpes simples. *Antiviral Res* 39(1):55–61.

Tragini E, Tubaro A, Melis S, & Galli L. (1985). Evidence from two classic irritation tests for an anti-inflammatory action of a natural extract, echinacina B. *Food and Chemical Toxicology* 23(2):317–319.

Ultee A, Gorris LG, & Smid EJ. (1998). Bactericidal activity of carvacrol towards the food-borne pathogen Bacillus cereus. *J Appl Microbiol* 85(2):211–218.

Vazqyue B, Avila G, Segura D, & Escalante B. (1996). Anti-inflammatory activity of extracts from Aloe vera gel. *J Ethnopharmacol* 55(1):69–75.

Visalyaputra S, Petchpaisit N, Somcharoen K, & Choavaratana R. (1998). The efficacy of ginger root in the prevention of postoperative nausea and vomiting after outpatient gynaecological laparoscopy. *Anesthesia* 53(5):506–510.

Vogel G. (1980). Silymarin, das antiheptotoxische wirkprinzip aus silybum marianum L. Gaertn., als antagonist der phalloidin-wirkung. *Arzneimittel-Forschung* 18:1063–1064.

von Schonfeld J, Weisbrod B, & Muller MK. (1997). Silibinin, a plant extract with antioxidant and membrane stabilizing properties, protects exocrine pancreas from cyclosporin A toxicity. *Cell Mol Life Sci* 53(11-12):917–920.

Wacker A, & Hilbig A. (1978). Virus inhibition by echinacea purpurea. *Planta Medica* 33:89–102.

Wang BX, Cui JC, Lui AJ, & Wu SK. (1983). Studies in the anti-fatigue effect of the saponins of stems and leaves of panax ginseng. *Journal of Traditional Chinese Medicine* 3(2):89–94. *Cancer Research* 58(9):1920–1929.

Wirth S. (1998). *Integrative Medicine, a Balanced Account of the Data.* Ukiah, CA: Creative Logic Co.

Xi X, Mukhtar H, & Agarwal R. (1997). Novel cancer chemopreventive effects of a flavonoid antioxidant Silyman: inhibition of an RNA expression of an endogenous tumor promoter TNF alpha. *Biochem Biophys Res Commun* 239(1):334–339.

Yasukawa K, Akihisa T, Oinuma H, Kaminaga T, Kanno H, Kasahara Y, Tamura T, Kumaki K, Yamanouchi S, & Takido M. (1996). Inhibitory effect of taraxastane-type triterpenes on tumor promotion by 12-0-tetradecanylphorbol-13-acetate in two-stage carcinogenesis in mouse skin. *Oncology* 53(4):341–344.

Yin MC, & Cheng WS. (1998). Inhibition of Aspergillus niger and Aspergillus flavus by some herbs and spices. *J Food Prot* 61(1):123–125.

Yoshida H, Iwata N, Katsuzaki H, Nagawana R, Ishikawa K, Fukuda H, Fujino T, & Suzuki A. (1998). Antimicrobal activity of a compound isolated from an oil-macerated garlic extract. *Biosci Biotechnol Biochem* 62(5):1014–1017.

You KM, Son KH, Chang HW, Kang SS, & Kim HP. (1998). Vitexicarpin, a flavonoid from the fruits of Vitex rotundifolia, inhibits mouse lymphocyte proliferation and growth of cell lines in vitro. *Planta Med* 64:546–550.

Zhao BL, Li XJ, Liu GT, Jia WY, & Xin WJ. (1990). Acavenging effect of schizandrins on active oxygen radicals. *Cell Biol Int Rep* 14(2):99–109.

Zi X, Grasso AW, Kung HJ, & Agarwal R. (1998). A flavaonoid antioxidant, silymarin, inhibits activation of erB1 signaling and induces cyclin-dependent kinase inhibitors, G1 arrest, and anti-carcenogenic effects in human prostate DU145 cells. *Cancer Res* 58(9):1920–1929.

Zi X, Feyes DK, & Agarwal R. (1998). Anticarcinogenic effect of flavonoid antioxidant, silymarin, in human breast cancer cells MDA-MB 468: induction of G1 arrest through an increase in Cip1/p21 concomittant with a decrease in kinase activity of cyclin-dependent kinases and associated cyclins. *Clin Cancer Res* 4(4):1055–1064.

Zou QZ, Bi RG, Li JM, Feng JB, Yu AM, Chan HP, & Zhen MX. (1989). Effect of motherwort on blood hyperviscosity. *Am J Chin Med* 17(1–2):65–70.

11

AROMATHERAPY

Aromatherapy is the use of essential plant oils to influence body, mind, or spirit (Kusmirek, 1992). The distillation of plant oils has a 5,000-year history. The Egyptians used the essential oils of myrrh, cedarwood, cinnamon, sandalwood, thyme, and elemi to embalm their dead. Incense was used to help heighten spiritual experiences by deepening meditation and purifying the spirit. The Babylonians, Hindus, Chinese, Japanese, Assyrians, ancient Africans, Greeks, Romans, and Native American shamans all used essential oils. The modern revival of their use began during the 1920s when Gattefosse, a French chemist and perfumer, coined the term aromatherapy (Wilson, 1995; Stevensen, 1996).

SCIENTIFIC BASIS

The liquid gas chromatograph is used to analyze chemical components of essential oils, yielding internationally accepted levels. The instrument can demonstrate the proportions of each oil compound, and distinguish between geographical locations, life-cycle stage at harvesting, and plant varieties (Vickers, 1996).

Essential oils are a mixture of over 100 organic compounds. According to Stevensen (1996) their therapeutic action includes aldehydes (calmants, anti-infectives), esters (antispasmodic, calmants, antifungicidal), ketones (calmants, mucolitics, litholitics, cicatrisings), coumarins (balancing, calming), lactones (balancing, calmants), sesquiterpenes (anti-allergics, antihistamines), acids/aromatic aldehydes (immunostimulants, anti-infectives), oxides (expectorants, antiparasitics), C10 terpenes (antiseptics, cortisonelike actions), phenols/C10 alcohols, aromatic aldehydes (anti-infectives, immunostimulants), C15 and C20 alcohols (estrogenlike actions), and phenyl methyl ethers (anti-infectives, antispasmodics).

The antimicrobial actions of essential oils have been the most widely researched. Thyme, sage, tarragon, geraniol, eugenol, menthol, and citral have all been shown to have high antibacterial activity (Panizzi, Flamini, Cioni, & Morelli, 1993; Moleyar & Narasimham, 1992; Stevensen, 1996). Animal studies showed that sandalwood, rose, and lavender had sedative effects on mice (Buchbauer, 1991; Price, 1995). Torri and colleagues (1988) demonstrated that inhalation of essential oils affects brain wave activity. Jasmine, clove, basil, peppermint, rose, and ylang ylang were identified as stimulating oils. Lavender, chamomile, lemon, marjoram, and sandalwood showed relaxing qualities.

Some randomized studies also show statistically significant results for essential oils. In a controlled trial with 100 post-cardiac surgery adults in intensive care, those who received a foot massage with nervoli citrus oil showed reduced anxiety compared to those massaged with plain vegetable oil (Stevensen, 1994). Compared to a non-chammomile massage, a massage with chamomile essential oil brought statistically significant results on the Rotterdam Symptom Checklist and the State-trait anxiety inventory (Wilkinson, 1995) in a study of 51 patients attending a center for palliative care.

HOW ESSENTIAL OILS WORK

Essential oils probably work on several levels. Smell may be the most complex and least understood method by which essential oils affect individuals. When a bottle of essential oil is opened, volatile aromatic molecules permeate the air. On inhalation, the molecules enter the nostrils, drift upward into the olfactory receptacles in the nose, where the cilia detect the scent and nerve cells relay the information to the limbic system in the brain. There, odors can trigger memories, emotions, immune responses, and the production of hormones that govern appetite, insulin production, metabolism, stress levels, sex drive, body temperature, and conscious thought (Wilson, 1995).

Essential oils also work through the skin by stimulating circulation and soothing inflamed or irritated cells. Some oils soothe sore muscles, release muscle spasms, and reduce muscular tension. It may be that once oil molecules penetrate the skin, they travel to internal organs and the lymphatic system to affect the immune system (Wilson, 1995).

PURCHASING QUALITY ESSENTIAL OILS

Not all essential oils are of equal quality. One easy way to tell the quality of an oil is the paper test. When a drop of essential oil is placed on a piece of paper, it evaporates, leaving no trace. Essential oils in carrier oils leave an oily spot (Wilson, 1995).

METHODS OF ADMINISTRATION

Skin Administration

Once a quality essential oil has been purchased, it is diluted in a carrier oil. Any vegetable oil will work, but some are preferable. Essential oils in the pure state are too concentrated to be used directly on the skin. They must be mixed with carrier or base oils before being massaged into the skin. Table 11.1 provides information on carrier or base oils used for dilution (Worwood, 1991).

Up to a maximum of 5 drops are used to each teaspoon of base oil. A brown glass bottle (with the volume imprinted on the bottom) can be purchased from a pharmacy. Base oil is measured, essential oil added and mixed by turning the bottle upside down several times. A teaspoon of mixed oils is usually adequate for massage (Worwood, 1991).

Inhalant Administration

For inhalant administration, 1 drop of essential oil is placed in a tissue or handkerchief and sniffed as needed (Worwood, 1991).

Table 11.1   Base Oils for Essential Oils

Base Oil	Uses	Dilution
Almond, Sweet	all skin types; itching, soreness, inflammation, dryness	100%
Apricot	all skin types; sensitive and aging skin	100%
Avocado, Pear	all skin types, especially dry and dehydrated, eczema	10%
Borage Seed	all skin types; regenerate and stimulate	10%
Carrot	reduces scarring, premature aging, itching, drying, psoriasis, eczema	10%
Evening Primrose	eczema, psoriasis	10%
Hazelnut	all skin types; astringent	100%
Jojoba	all skin types; inflammation, psoriasis, eczema, hair	10%
Olive	soothes rheumatic conditions	10%
Sesame	all skin types; psoriasis, eczema	10%
Soya Bean	all skin types	100%
Sunflower	all skin types	100%
Wheatgerm	all skin types; eczema, psoriasis, aging skin	10%

Bath Administration

For bath administration, essential oil is added to running bath water. The bathroom door is closed so vapors do not escape. The individual soaks for at least 10 minutes, breathing deeply.

Room Administration

Room administration includes diffusers, humidifiers, room sprays, and water bowls. A diffuser made especially for essential oils is suggested. It should have a bowl section that is nonporous so it can be wiped clean.

GUIDELINES FOR USING ESSENTIAL OILS

Guidelines for using essential oils include:

1. Buy essential oil from reliable sources that guarantee the purity of their oils.
2. Keep essential oils tightly capped away from sun and heat, in dark glass bottles.
3. Always dilute essential oils in a carrier oil before applying to the body.
4. Drop the oils from a dropper into a clean container for blending.
5. Do not exceed the number of recommended drops of an essential oil.
6. Avoiding shaking a bottle of essential oil. To mix, tip the bottle upside down a number of times.
7. Trust the nose. If the user dislikes the smell, avoid that essential oil.
8. Inhale essential oils for short periods and diffuse for only 5 to 10 minutes at a time.
9. Check with a qualified aromatherapist as needed.

Table 11.2 suggests essential oils for specific conditions.
Table 11.3 provides informations on cautions to take when using essential oils.

Table 11.2 Suggested Essential Oils for Specific Conditions/Effects

Condition	Suggested Essential Oils
Aborted fetus	geranium or Roman chamomile or rose or palmarosa or frankincense
Acceptance, lack of	ginger or juniper
Addiction, drug	rose or orange or nutmeg or eucalyptus or juniper or lime or sweet marjoram or basil

(continued)

Table 11.2   *(continued)*

	or peppermint or grapefruit or fennel or parsley or sandalwood
Agitation	juniper
Allergies	melissa or garlic
Amnesia	rose
Anger	Spanish sage or ylang ylang or sandalwood or petitgrain or oregano or myrtle or chamomile (German) or chamomile (Roman) or cypress or garlic (promotes forgiveness) or lavender or linden
Anorexia Nervosa	bay or carrot seed
Anxiety	rosewood or verbena or geranium or German chamomile or marjoram or lavender or Spanish sage or ylang ylang or vetivert or violet or patchouli or oregano or neroli or bergamot or chamomile (Roman) or coriander or frankincense or geranium or mandarin or lavender or lime
Anxiety and fear massage oil	bergamot (7 drops), geranium (3 drops), clary sage (4 drops)*
Apathy	garlic or jasmine or lime
Appetite stimulant	nutmeg or myrrh or bay or bergamot or caraway or carrot seed or ginger or mandarin
Appetite suppressant	patchouli
Arthritis	Spanish sage or vetivert or yarrow or pine or benzoin or bergamot or cajuput or chamomile (Roman) or clove or fir or eucalyptus or geranium or lemon or thyme or lavender
Rheumatoid arthritis massage oil	lavender (10 drops), eucalyptus (10 drops), peppermint (19 drops), thyme (5 drops)*
Osteoarthritis massage oil	ginger (10 drops), basil (5 drops), marjoram (10 drops)*
Asthma	tea tree or rosemary or rose or peppermint or oregano or niaouli or melissa or basil or cajuput or clary sage or cypress or fennel or fir (acute) or lime
Aura balancing	sandalwood or peppermint or petitgrain
Aura cleansing	pine or rose or Spanish sage or tea tree or peppermint or cloves or fir or lime or mandarin
Aura energizes	ginger

Table 11.2 *(continued)*

Aura protection	vetivert
Aura revitalizing	orange
Aura, reform after illness or accident	neroli
Aura, strengthens and recharges	caraway
Bad breath	parsley
Bladder	parsley
Blood clotting	garlic (thins blood)
Breast milk, increases	caraway or dill or fennel or geranium or clary sage
Breathing/expands chest	cinnamon
Breathing, slows	frankincense
Bruising	hyssop
Burns	chamomile (German) or frankincense or lavender or marigold
Catarrh	red thyme or niaouli or lime or linden
Cell destruction	lavender
Centers	bergamot
Chakras	myrrh (opens base chakra, allows life force energy to flow into kidneys, polarizes base and crown chakras) or camphor (opens base chakra) or star anise (crown chakra) or dill (crown chakra) or frankincense (crown chakra)
Childbirth, eases	cinnamon or dill
Chills	bergamot or coriander or ginger
Cholesterol	orange
Circulatory conditions	coriander or yarrow or Spanish sage or vetivert or rosemary or rose or pine or bergamot or caraway or cinnamon or ginger or lemon or lemongrass
Circulation, localized	niaouli
Circulation, stimulates	cumin or geranium or lime
Massage oil (massage in the direction of the heart)	geranium (10 drops), peppermint (5 drops), rose (10 drops), patchouli (5 drops)*
Collagen formation	orange
Colic	peppermint or parsley or oregano or cardamom or coriander or ginger
Concentration	cardamom or eucalyptus

(continued)

Table 11.2   *(continued)*

Conception	melissa
Congestion, general	cumin
Congestion, nasal	thyme, red
Congestion, lungs and respiratory tract	basil
Constipation	yarrow or parsley or oregano or dill or sweet marjoram
Coughs	tea tree or red thyme or sandalwood or pimento or oregano or niaouli or melissa or cajuput or ginger or jasmine or lemon
Cramping	verbena or yarrow or peppermint or cardamom or clary sage or dill or ginger or sweet marjoram
Foot bath for leg cramps	geranium (5 drops), lavender (10 drops), cypress (2 drops) in a bowl of hot, not boiling, water
Creative blocks	cloves or fennel or geranium
Cuts	pine
Cystitis	tea tree or niaouli or bergamot or juniper or sage or cypress
Massage hips, lower back, and abdomen daily	sage (5 drops), oregano (5 drops), niaouli (20 drops)*
Delusions	clary sage
Dementia	lavender or lime
Depression	nutmeg or bergamot or clove or Spanish sage or red thyme or verbena or ylang ylang or rose or patchouli or nutmeg or celery or chamomile (Roman) or cinnamon or citronella or clary sage or geranium or coriander or cypress or eucalyptus or grapefruit or jasmine or lime
Depression, post-natal	clary sage or neroli or grapefruit or rose or angelica or mandarin
Diabetes	eucalyptus or peppermint or geranium or cypress or ginger or hyssop
Body massage	lavender (3 drops), geranium (12 drops) eucalyptus (5 drops), peppermint (5 drops), ginger (5 drops)*
Diarrhea	sandalwood or clove or coriander or mandarin
Digestion	petitgrain or parsley or palmarosa or orange or nutmeg or bergamot (animal fats) or car-

Table 11.2 *(continued)*

	rot seed or chamomile (German) or cinnamon (sluggish) or citronella or coriander or cumin or dill or lavender or lemon (stomach acidity) or mandarin
Dysentery	melissa
Earache	bay or hyssop
Edema, body rub	ginger (3 drops), cypress (2 drops), lavender (2 drops)*
Endometriosis	
Alternate hot and cold waist-deep baths	geranium (10 drops), rose (5 drops), cypress (2 drops), nutmeg (10 drops), clary sage (8 drops)
and	
Twice daily hip and abdominal massage	clary sage (5 drops), rose (5 drops), geranium (10 drops), nutmeg (10 drops)*
Energy blocks	peppermint (heart to crown), sandalwood (base to crown), patchouli (integrates base and crown), verbena (creates spiritual space), yarrow (third eye), ylang ylang (contentment/acceptance)
Eyes	rose or fennel
Fainting/vertigo	peppermint
Fatigue/exhaustion	white thyme or lavender or Spanish sage or violet or rosemary or rose or pine or pimento or patchouli or oregano or nutmeg or fir (mental) or ginger
Foot bath	4–5 drops in a bowl of hot, but not scalding water
Body rub	lavender (10 drops), grapefruit (10 drops), coriander (10 drops)*
Fear	
of change	lavender
of death	juniper
Fever/flu	yarrow or peppermint or palmarosa or niaouli or angelica or basil or benzoin or bergamot or cajuput or celery (fever) or coriander or ginger or grapefruit or juniper or lemon or lime or linden
Flatulence	yarrow or oregano or melissa or angelica or cardamom or clary sage or coriander or dill or ginger or lavender or sweet marjoram

(continued)

Table 11.2   *(continued)*

Fungal infection	tea tree or myrrh or lemongrass (athlete's foot)
Gallbladder	carrot seed (tonic) or fennel or garlic
Gallstones	bergamot or eucalyptus
Gastro-enteritis	lemongrass
Genito-Urinary Problems	cedarwood
Gout	violet or pine or juniper
Grief	cypress or chamomile (Roman) or fir or grapefruit (emotional or mental violence) or hyssop or linden or sweet marjoram
Grounding	red thyme or vetivert or benzoin or celery or fir (while allowing love to flow) or jasmine
Guilt	nutmeg
Hay fever	eucalyptus
Headaches	lime or peppermint or Spanish sage or violet or rosemary or peppermint or pimento or oregano or cardamom or chamomile (tension) or clary sage or dill or eucalyptus or grapefruit or linden (migraines)
Heart	rose or neroli or aniseed or coriander or geranium or lavender or marigold
Massage front of torso in clockwise direction	geranium (14 drops), hyssop (4 drops), peppermint (4 drops), rosemary (8 drops)*
Heartburn	cardamom
Hemorrhoids	juniper
Herpes	rose
Hormonal imbalance	Spanish sage or fennel
Hyperactivity	lavender
Hypertension	yarrow or ylang ylang or rose or camphor or celery or clary sage or garlic or lavender
Hypotension	rosemary or rose or hyssop
Hypothermia	cinnamon
Hysteria	oregano or basil or bergamot or lavender or linden
Impotence	aniseed
Immune system	lavender or rosewood or myrtle or bergamot or fir or lime
Incontinence	cypress
Indigestion	star anise or Spanish sage or verbena or melissa or yarrow or peppermint or angelica

Table 11.2 *(continued)*

	or cardamom or celery or clove or ginger or lemongrass
Infection, chest	sweet marjoram
Infection, mouth	bergamot
Infection, throat	white thyme
Infection, viral	thyme, red or bay or bergamot or cajuput or eucalyptus or juniper
Infection, bacterial	tea tree or nutmeg or bergamot or garlic or juniper or eucalyptus
Infection with fever	lemongrass
Infertility	
Female	cypress or geranium or clary sage or thyme or nutmeg or Roman chamomile or coriander
Male	thyme or basil or cumin or cedarwood or sage or clary sage or vetiver
Inflammation	marigold or yarrow or violet or rose or bay or chamomile (Roman) or clary sage or hyssop or marigold
Insomnia	linden blossom or lavender or violet or sandalwood or oregano or neroli or chamomile (German and Roman) or dill or lavender or linden
Intestines, calms	neroli
Intestines, cleanses	basil
Intestines/parasites	niaouli or clove
Intestinal spasm	clove
Irritability	cardamom
Joints, stiff	oregano or bergamot
Joints, swollen	sweet marjoram
Kidneys	violet or parsley or basil or clove or garlic (cleanses) or linden
Kidney stones	bergamot
Laryngitis	red thyme or cajuput or jasmine
Lethargy	cloves or citronella or jasmine
Liver	rose or verbena or violet or rosemary or peppermint or bay or carrot seed (tonic) or celery or cumin or eucalyptus or linden
Lymphatic cleanser	angelica or bergamot or frankincense or garlic

(continued)

Table 11.2   *(continued)*

Memory/clear thought	patchouli or white thyme or rosemary or cloves or red thyme or citronella or coriander or cypress or ginger
Menopause	neroli or geranium or sage or nutmeg or red thyme or jasmine
Hot flashes massage oil	clary sage (10 drops), geranium (11 drops), lemon (7 drops), sage (2 drops)*
Mood swings	lavender or patchouli or cypress or linden
Mouth sores	cloves or lime
Muscular aches	rosemary or nutmeg or bergamot or eucalyptus or fir or lemongrass
Muscular spasms	petitgrain or carrot seed or cinnamon or jasmine or lavender
Nausea	peppermint or star anise or rosemary or rose or pimento or basil or ginger or lavender or coriander or fennel
Nosebleeds	cypress
Obsessiveness	clary sage or sandalwood or juniper
Osteoporosis	
Bath	use up to a total of 4 drops total of 1–3 of the following: ginger, chamomile (German), rosemary, fennel, lemon, thyme, hyssop
Massage most susceptible joints	ginger (10 drops), nutmeg (7 drops), carrot (5 drops), Roman chamomile (8 drops)
Overweight	patchouli or juniper or mandarin
Pain	birch or pine or clove or violet or rose or pimento or chamomile (Roman) or clove (general and during childbirth) or clary sage (labor) or ginger or hyssop
Pain, back	sweet marjoram
Pain, labor	jasmine
Pancreas, stimulates	lemon
Paranoia	clary sage
Phobias	rosemary or oregano or linden
PMS/menstrual problems	rose or star anise or clary sage or parsley or neroli or melissa or cardamom or carrot seed or chamomile (German and Roman) (promotes menstruation) or frankincense (heavy periods) or geranium or grapefruit (PMS) or lavender (scant and painful periods) or marigold or fennel

Table 11.2 *(continued)*

Purpose, lack of	cinnamon
Raynaud's Disease	
Massage oil	nutmeg (15 drops), lavender (5 drops), geranium (10 drops)*
Bath	6–8 drops of the above blended
Recurring dreams	sandalwood
Reproductive problems	carrot or bay laurel or vetivert or carrot seed
Resentment	garlic (promotes forgiveness) or lemon
Respiratory conditions	pine or star anise or hyssop or clove or sandlewood or tea tree or violet or niaouli or rosemary or oregano or orange or myrtle or myrrh or benzoin or caraway or cedarwood (expectorant) or fennel or fir or frankincense or ginger or lavender or lime
Restlessness	juniper
Self-esteem, low	peppermint or myrtle or myrrh or aniseed or basil or citronella or clary sage or dill or grapefruit
Self-hate	fennel
Sexual blocks	sandalwood or rosewood or rose or nutmeg or myrtle or cardamom or celery (restores libido) or clary sage or cumin or jasmine
Shock	tea tree or verbena or melissa or bergamot
Sinusitis	tea tree or red thyme or cajuput or ginger
Skin	Spanish sage or verbena or vetivert or yarrow or sandalwood or rose or pine or petitgrain or patchouli or palmarosa or myrrh (wrinkles) or benzoin (clears, makes glow) or chamomile (German) or fennel or hyssop or lavender or lemongrass
Sore throat	thyme, red or star anise or bergamot or cajuput or ginger
Spleen	cloves or coriander
Sprains	vetivert or bergamot or chamomile (Roman)
Stomach, warms	coriander
Stress	carrot or orange or neroli or chamomile (Roman) or lemongrass or sweet marjoram
Stretch marks/scars/thread veins	neroli
Toothache	hyssop
Throat, sore	caraway or geranium or lemon or lime

(continued)

Table 11.2 *(continued)*

Thyroid dysfunction	garlic
Tissue healing	niaouli
Tonsilitis	red thyme or bergamot or geranium
Trapped feeling	fir
Trauma	white thyme or cajuput (after emotional, mental or psychic attack)
Trauma, childhood	nutmeg
Tumors, cancerous	hyssop
Ulcers	cloves or geranium
Urinary conditions	myrtle
Uterine conditions	rose or jasmine or melissa or geranium
Uterine hemorrhage	frankincense
Vaginitis	tea tree
Varicose veins	
Grab ankle and massage gently up leg once with one hand	geranium (10 drops), cypress (10 drops), lemon (5 drops), peppermint (5 drops)*
Foot baths	Soak feet 5 minutes in a bowl of cold water with 2 drops lavender followed by soaking in a bowl of warm water with 2 drops of geranium.
Vomiting	cardamom or lavender
Warts	lime or lavender or cypress
Water balance (restores)	palmarosa or grapefruit or mandarin
Water retention	patchouli or celery or fennel or lemon or peppermint
Weakness	fennel
Wounds/sores	myrrh or yarrow or tea tree or frankincense or geranium or hyssop or juniper

*Diluted in 2 tablespoons base oil.
Excerpted from: *Colour Scents, Healing with Colour and Aroma* by S. Chizzari, Cambridge: CW Daniel; *Essential Oils and Aromatherapy* by V.A. Worwood, San Rafael: New World Library.

Table 11.3   Cautions When Using Essential Oils

Cautions	Oils
Avoid during pregnancy	angelica, aniseed, basil, bay, camphor, carrot seed, cedarwood, celery, citronella, Clary sage, cumin, cypress, dill, fennel, geranium, hyssop, marigold, marjoram, me-

Table 11.3 *(continued)*

Cautions	Oils
	lissa, myrrh, nutmeg, jasmine, lavender, oregano, parsley, rose, rosemary, sage, thyme, yarrow
Avoid when breastfeeding	garlic
Avoid with diabetes	angelica
Avoid with eczema	garlic
Avoid with fiery temperaments	garlic
Avoid with hypertension	eucalyptus, hyssop, rose, rosemary, thyme
Avoid with hypotension	lavender
Avoid if photosensitive	bergamot, angelica, ginger, lemon, mandarin, verbena
Avoid if have allergies	star anise
Avoid if epileptic	camphor, eucalyptus, fennel, hyssop, rose, rosemary
Can cause convulsions	cinnamon
Can be toxic and hallucinogenic	parsley, nutmeg
Can cause dermatitis	aniseed, basil
Can irritate mucus membranes at high doses	myrtle, pimento (use at 1%)
Can be toxic	sandalwood, sage (adverse effect on CNS)
Check for skin allergies	juniper
Headaches and nausea in large doses	benzoin
May cause drowsiness	marjoram, neroli, sandalwood
May irritate sensitive skin	cajuput, caraway, cedarwood, clove, citronella, cumin, lemon, lime, linden, melissa, orange, peppermint, pine, tea tree
Narcotic in large doses	aniseed
Phototoxic	ginger, mandarin, orange, verbena
Phototoxic in sun	bergamot
Possible sensitization	niaouli
Use in 1% dilution	birch, cinnamon, lemongrass
Stupefying in large doses	coriander
Use in low dosage	thyme
Use in moderation, can cause headache/ nausea	ylang ylang

Source: Extracted from: *Colour Scents, Healing with Colour and Aroma* by Suzy Chiazzari, Cambridge: C.W. Daniel Company Ltd, 1998.

REFERENCES

Buchbauer G. (1991). Aromatherapy: Evidence for the sedative effects of the essential oil of lavender after inhalation. *Zeitschrift Fur Naturforschung* 46:1067–1072.

Kusmirek J. (1992). Perspectives in aromatherapy. In Van Toller S, Dodd GH (Eds.), *Fragrance: The Psychology and Biology of Perfume*. Barking: Elsevier Science Pub. Ltd.

Moleyar V, & Narasimham P. (1992). Antibacterial activity of essential oil components. *Int J Food Microbiol* 16(4):337–342.

Panizzi L, Flamini G, Cioni PL, & Morelli I. (1993). Composition and antimicrobial properties of essential oils of four Mediterranean Lamiaceae. *J Ethnopharmacol* 39(3):167–170.

Price S. (1995). *Aromatherapy for Health Care Professionals*. Edinburgh: Churchill Livingstone.

Stevensen CJ. (1994). The psychophysiological effects of aromatherapy massage following cardiac surgery. *Complementary Ther Med* 2:27–35.

Stevensen CJ. (1996). Aromatherapy. In Micozzi MS (Ed.), *Fundamentals of Complementary and Alternative Medicine* (pp. 137–148). New York: Churchill Livingstone.

Torri S, Fukuda H, & Kanemoto H. (1988). Continent negative variation (CNV) and the psychological effects of odour. In Van Toller S, Dodd GH (Eds.), *Perfumery: The Psychology and Biology of Fragrance* (pp. 107–121). London: Chapman and Hall.

Vickers A. (1996). *Massage and Aromatherapy: A Guide for Health Professionals*. London: Chapman Hall.

Wilkinson S. (1995). Aromatherapy and massage in palliative care. *International J Palliative Nursing* 1(1):21–30.

Wilson R. (1995). *Aromatherapy*. Garden City Park, NY: Avery Publishing Group.

Worwood VA. (1991). *The Complete Book of Essential Oils & Aromatherapy*. San Rafael, CA: New World Library.

B

Healing Systems

12

AYURVEDA

Ayurveda is a word of Sanskrit origin that means daily living (ayus) with knowledge (vid). The story of Ayurveda began some 5,000 years ago in India. A group of holy men known as the Rishis compiled texts of Hindu spirituality and philosophy into Vedas. There are four main branches of Vedic science including yoga, self-knowledge, Vedic astrology, and Ayurveda. The practice of following these texts for physical healing, diet, herbs, and massage or bodywork, comprises Ayurvedic practice.

Health is not the ultimate goal, but is believed to be important for spiritual growth. The practice is holistic, integrating body, mind, and spirit with the forces of nature. Five elements—earth, fire, air, water, and space—combine and give rise to prana (energy) that regulates the body through doshas (or forces) called vata, pitta, and kapha (Zwolski, 1999; Collinge, 1996). The doshas are basic metabolic principles that govern the psychophysiological structure and process.

THE DOSHAS: VATA DISPERSES

Vata is a combination of air and space. The Vata principle guides the flow of information and matter, organizing the nervous system, and moves nourishment in and out of the cells. Because vata governs the nervous system, it is the dosha most easily imbalanced by stress. The fast-paced hectic lifestyle of Western society results in vata imbalances on a massive scale. Vata is associated with the digestive, respiratory, cardiovascular, reproductive/sexual, and elimination systems. The bones and joints are also served by vata. In a health state, vata is expressed as creativity, exuberance, and joy. When excess vata exists, vata imbalance occurs and can be observed as lightness, excess quickness, butterflies in the stomach, vertigo, loneliness, fearfulness, insomnia, or emptiness. When not enough vata exists, dry skin and nails, and other dry conditions abound: constipation, osteoarthritis, osteoporosis, endometriosis, flatulence, sciatica, light-headedness, dizziness and lack of coordination, or general lack of feeling grounded (Lonsdorf, Butler, & Brown, 1993; Collinge, 1996). Vaginal dryness, emotional mood swings, and insomnia of menopause all represent Vata dosha imbalance (Lonsdorf et al., 1993).

119

People who are primarily vata worry frequently, have difficulty falling asleep or having a sound night's sleep, do not memorize easily or remember what was memorized, are enthusiastic and vivacious, perform activities quickly, and may disperse a lot of energy, sometimes wastefully (Chopra, 1994). They often spend money easily and prefer an artistic or music-related life rather than a mainstream position. Conditions that can befall vata individuals include intestinal gas, lower back pain, sciatica, arthritis, neuralgia, paralysis, and/or nervous afflictions (Collinge, 1996). Causes may be related to excessive exercise, not enough rest, suppression of natural urges, overwork, fear, grief, worry, excessive raw food, overexposure to cold, fasting, and too many pungent foods.

Vata tends to increase with age for all doshas, making individuals drier, colder, and less tolerant of cold winters. All older people tend to do best in warm climates.

Vata time is early in the morning, starting at 2:00 a.m. and continuing on until 6:00 a.m., and again in the afternoon 2:00 to 6:00 p.m. Starting the day at or before 6:00 a.m. is associated with alertness, creativity, and action. More energy, creativity, and alertness will be available during the day and less effort will be required to be productive (Lonsdorf et al., 1993).

Vata season is mid-October to mid-February. It is a time to keep the head and neck warm as cold drafts can lead to cold, flu, cough, and related conditions. It is a time to avoid cold foods and drink.

THE DOSHAS: KAPHA ACCUMULATES

Kapha is a combination of earth and water. It commands the building of the body structure, including tissues, bones, strength, lubrication, and cohesive support. It is associated with mucus and fluid production. Imbalance (too little or too much) appears in the stomach, lymph system, lungs, mouth, and joints. When out of balance, the body's ability to deal with excess fluids can result in water retention, congestion, lethargy, or heaviness (Lonsdorf et al., 1993).

Kapha individuals are relaxed and take their time. They have a calm disposition and gain weight easily. They sleep like babies and are not easily ruffled under stress. All their body processes, including their digestive systems, work slowly, so they may feel heavy after eating. They can accumulate great wealth and make good middle managers. Dis-eases that plague kapha types are sinusitis, lung congestion, tonsilitis, fluid retention, and bronchitis. Causes may be related to sleeping during the day, lack of exercise, heavy food, milk products, and too many salty, sour, or sweet foods.

Kapha time is between 6:00 p.m. and 10:00 p.m. and is the ideal time to go to sleep because the deep calming influence of Kapha is available then. Also, less sleep may be required by going to bed before 10 p.m.

Kapha season is spring. It is a time to lighten the diet and increase exercise. The best time to exercise and wake up the body is during Kapha time at 6:00 a.m. to 10:00 a.m. or a 15-minute walk after dinner 6:00 p.m. to 10:00 p.m.

THE DOSHAS: PITTA TRANSFORMS

Pitta is a combination of water and fire. Pitta is a go-between for Vata and Kapha, conducting the transformation of energy and heat production. Pitta is responsible for digestive enzymes, hormonal system, heart, blood, liver, intestines, eyes, skin, and spleen. When excess heat occurs, there is an imbalance and inflammation, skin eruptions, ulcers, emotional irritability or temper appear. The hotflashes of menopause represent a Pitta imbalance (Lonsdorf et al., 1993). Early graying, excessive hot flashes during menopause, and stress-related heart attacks and heartburn are other signs of imbalance. Signs of excessive pitta are excessive hunger and thirst (Lansdorf et al., 1993).

Pitta individuals are precise, orderly, efficient, forceful, and strong-minded. They feel uncomfortable skipping a meal and can perspire easily. At work, they are engaged in transforming one thing into another, often as CEOs of corporations. They have fiery qualities: aggressiveness, a red face, and/or competitiveness. Because they are efficient, they budget their resources easily and improve their standard of living. When they fall ill, it is often due to liver and gallbladder disorders, peptic ulcers, inflammatory disease, skin disorders, gastritis, or hyperacidity. Causes of imbalance include anger, alcohol, salty, sour, or spicy foods, strong sunshine and the heat of summer, vinegar, and wine.

Pitta time is 10 p.m to 2 a.m. Sleeping during these hours aids digestion, while staying awake increases food cravings. Skin problems may be improved by going to bed before pitta time. Late-nighters can gradually shift their bedtime by going to bed first at midnight, then at 11 p.m. and so on.

Pitta season is mid-June to mid-October, a time for cool drinks and salads. But, too many tomatoes and cold drinks can lead to skin problems, urinary tract infections, other inflammatory conditions, and irritability. A remedy is to continue drinking warm drinks all through the season and resist eating too many tomatoes and shellfish (Lansdorf et al., 1993).

ASSESSING DOSHAS

Use Table 12.1 when assessing individuals in the Ayurvedic framework. If one column is 15 or more points higher than the others, that is the dominant constitutional type. Most people are a combination of two of the doshas, although one force usually predominates. It is possible to be a dual-dosha or even a tri-dosha (if all three column totals are within 0–10 points of each other).

TREATING DOSHA IMBALANCE

The accumulation of metabolic wastes from imbalanced digestion is related to many dis-eases: (1) underutilized carbohydrates contribute to diabetes and its complications; (2) excessive protein by-products can lead to urate crystals and

Table 12.1   Assessing Ayurvedic Type

Use the following rating system:

> 0 = does not describe the client
> 1 = describes the client a little
> 2 = describes the client well
> 3 = describes client almost perfectly

VATA

_____ Has dry, curly, hair that is full-bodied
_____ Performs activities quickly
_____ Skin is on the dry side
_____ Has difficulty memorizing and remembering what was memorized
_____ Is enthusiastic and vivacious by nature
_____ Is worried or anxious frequently
_____ Has difficulty falling asleep or having a sound night's sleep
_____ Varies from excessive to no interest in eating
_____ Prefers warm, moist and/or oily foods
_____ Eats quickly
_____ Is most sensitive to noise
_____ Is easy and impulsive with money
_____ Is thin, small, and dark
_____ Dislikes cold; comfortable in heat
_____ Is a light sleeper
_____ Energy level fluctuates, coming in waves
_____ Has difficulty gaining weight

Total Points: _____

PITTA

_____ Has blonde or reddish hair and complexion
_____ Skin is delicate, sensitive
_____ Is average sized
_____ Considers self to be efficient
_____ Has a forceful manner
_____ Perspires easily
_____ Becomes uncomfortable if a meal is delayed
_____ Is orderly and precise in activities
_____ Can push self too hard
_____ Hunger level is intense; needs regular meals
_____ Prefers cold foods
_____ Eats moderately fast
_____ Is quick tempered
_____ Reacts with irritation to stress
_____ Always finishes what is started
_____ Is determined
_____ Is most sensitive to bright light

Total Points: _____

Table 12.1 *(continued)*

KAPHA

_____ Has dark brown or black, thick, wavy, and shiny hair
_____ Is large-boned
_____ Skin is oily and smooth
_____ Gains weight easily and is slow to lose it
_____ Has a steady energy level
_____ Tolerates extremes well except dislikes damp cold
_____ Hunger level is usually low but can be driven by emotion
_____ Prefers warm, dry foods
_____ Reacts to stress with calm
_____ Sleeps deep and long and is slow to awaken
_____ Is most sensitive to strong odors
_____ Is even tempered and slow to anger
_____ Is slow to make friends, but always loyal
_____ Voice is soothing and rich with moments of silence
_____ Is methodical
_____ Characterized as easygoing
_____ Learns by associating new information with a memory

Total Points: _____

Dominant Dosha:
Dual-Dosha:
Tri-Dosha:

This figure is a compilation of information from Zucker (1995); Chopra (1994); and Lonsdorf, Butler, and Brown (1993).

gouty arthritis, osteoporosis and Alzheimer's disease; (3) an overconcentration of minerals can lead to kidney stones and many forms of arthritis; (4) Undigested fat can produce blockages leading to lipomas, cirrhosis of the liver, eye disease or hyperthyroidism, and obesity (Lansdorf et al., 1993).

In the Ayurvedic framework, food allergies may arise because food is not digested properly. The Vedic approach suggests that once digestion is improved and food is broken down into the proper simple molecules of sugar, protein, and fat, the body recognizes them as nutrition and not as an antigen needing an antibody (Lansdorf et al., 1993). For this reason, Ayurvedic treatments focus on eliminating toxic amas (obstructions to full psychophysiological functioning). Ama can be clogged arteries, the loneliness of a closed heart, writer's block, cellulite, doubt, or arthritic immobilization. Ama in the nervous system can represent undigested or unresolved mental and emotional difficulties, just as women with more (undigested) carcinogenic chemicals in their breasts are more apt to develop breast cancer. Overweight women are cautioned to eliminate wastes, not weight.

Ayurvedic treatment focuses on the digestive process as a major intervention area. This involves the physical food eaten as well as the food taken in mentally and emotionally when human beings read, watch television, have relationships, work, and so forth. Signs of digestive disorder include:

- coated tongue
- muscle and joint pain
- nasal congestion
- gas
- constipation
- frequent, loose stools
- rashes
- loss of appetite

Most individuals pay little attention to these signs and do not ask, "What happens when my food is not processed properly and wastes are not eliminated completely?" Ayurveda does ask this question and treats digestive and metabolic processes before illness can be detected by many allopathic methods.

AYURVEDIC NUTRITIONAL PRINCIPLES

Four principles are important in the Ayurvedic nutritional approach and can be taught to clients

1. Diet is a therapeutic modality and the central means of balancing the doshas.
2. How food is digested is as important as what is ingested.
3. Different individuals require different foods; Western nutritional recommendations tend to be universal without taking into account different metabolic rates.
4. The taste of food is nutritionally important, not just an extra; American meals often underrepresent bitter, pungent, and astringent tastes and overrepresent salty and sweet tastes. In the Ayurvedic method, 6 tastes are believed to be important.

THE SIX TASTES

For an ideal menu of nutrients to balance the doshas, clients can be counseled to include all 6 tastes. They can be told that cravings may be born out of skewing the diet toward sweet, salty, and sour, as is common in Western countries. The tendency to snack and not feel completely satisfied can be explained by describing the 6 tastes and their importance at every meal (Lansdorf et al., 1993; Collinge, 1996). Examples of each taste follow.

1. *Sweet*: sugar, milk, butter, rice, bread, pasta, and grains
2. *Pungent*: spicy foods, jalapeno peppers, ginger root, cayenne, cumin
3. *Bitter*: spinach and other green leafy vegetables, turmeric
4. *Astringent*: dried beans, bean soups, and green leafy vegetables, lentils, pomegranate
5. *Sour*: yogurt, lemon, grapefruit, and aged cheese
6. *Salty*: salt or any salty food

CASE STUDY

Harriet was a forty-year-old lawyer with three young children. She had battled over-weight since her early twenties and was never able to take off the weight she gained during her pregnancies. Finally, desperate, she started a strict low-fat diet and lost 60 pounds. For three months, she kept the weight off, by eating no more than 1,300 calories a day. However, she did not have menstrual periods anymore, she had developed dry skin and hair, and was irritable and cranky. Then she started to gain weight on the 1,300 calories and began to binge on ice cream and candy bars. She gained back the 60 pounds and 20 more.

She consulted an Ayurvedic practitioner and began to focus on eliminating ama (the blockages to adequate digestion). She was told to focus on adding more foods that were good for her rather than taking away other foods. The binge behavior ended and she started to slowly lose weight. She had a menstrual period and felt a tremendous feeling of relief. Also, rather than feeling miserable and deprived, she started to feel at peace.

GENERAL EATING PRINCIPLES FOR ALL DOSHAS

The following Ayurvedic principles are focused on improving digestion, including appropriate waste elimination (Lonsdorf et al., 1993), and can be incorporated into printed materials given to clients:

1. Make lunch the heaviest meal of the day when digestive power is at its height and there is less likelihood of gaining weight; be sure to include all 6 tastes.
2. Only eat while seated, preferably in a settled environment, and allow at least 20 minutes to eat.
3. Eat to three-fourths capacity, only to the point of satisfaction, not fullness.
4. Allow 3 to 6 hours between meals, avoiding eating until the previous meal has been digested.
5. Eat lightly when stressed or ill.
6. Avoid ice-cold beverages and foods; they reduce the efficiency of the digestive enzymes.
7. Sip warm water with meals and throughout the day to aid digestion.
8. Eat food hot or at least warm.
9. Eat at the same time every day.

10. Prepare foods from scratch to ensure purity and freshness of ingredients; avoid eating leftovers by making smaller quantities; cook foods well and insure the color, smell, taste, and texture are pleasing.
11. Cook in a pleasant environment; cooking tastes best and nourishes best when prepared with love.
12. Eat foods that are chemical-free and fresh.
13. Eat a light, early dinner (no later than 6 p.m. or 7 p.m.) and only have liquids after 8 p.m. Monitor sleep and arousal patterns after the meal to judge digestion and modify dinner accordingly.
14. Avoid yogurt, cheese, cottage cheese, and cultured buttermilk after sunset.
15. Avoid heating or cooking with honey.

In addition to incorporating these principles into lifestyle, the following additional principles are suggested for each of the doshas.

VATA IMBALANCE TREATMENT

Clients can be treated for vata imbalance by taking the following actions (Lonsdorf et al., 1993; Collinge, 1996):

1. Obtain adequate rest, preferably on a soft bed, by taking valerian root at night to promote calm sleep.
2. Attain regularity in all things.
3. Have a sesame oil massage to help eliminate toxins and calm the mind/body.
4. Stay warm.
5. Be in the company of warmhearted people.
6. Meditate daily to improve general well-being, reduce stress, and listen to the body's wisdom (see: meditation).
7. Calm the mind through alternate nostril breathing (see: breathing).
8. Eat warm, cooked foods.
9. Avoid cold foods and drinks.
10. Practice yoga postures daily.
11. Avoid large amounts of salads and raw vegetables.
12. Eat more: rice; wheat; all dairy products; molasses, honey, all oils; sweet fruits: grapes, cherries, peaches, melons, avocado, coconut, bananas, sweet oranges, sweet pineapples, sweet plums, sweet berries, mangoes, fresh figs, dates, apricots, stewed fruits; well-cooked vegetables: beets, carrots, asparagus, cucumber, sweet potatoes; all nuts; black pepper (in small quantity), cinnamon, cardamom, cumin, ginger, salt, clove, mustard seeds; chicken, turkey, and seafood.
13. Eat fewer: dry foods; cold or iced foods and drinks; pungent, bitter, or astringent foods; barley, corn, millet, buckwheat, rye, and oats; dried fruits, uncooked apples or pears, pomegranate, cranberries.

Overall: Favor sweet, sour, salty, heavy, oily, hot foods, and avoid pungent, bitter, astringent, light, dry, cold foods

PITTA IMBALANCE TREATMENT

Treat pitta imbalance by (Lansdorf et al., 1993; Collinge, 1996) teaching clients to:

1. Avoid overscheduling and overworking.
2. Eat meals on time, especially lunch.
3. Eat more cool foods and drinks, foods with sweet, bitter and astringent tastes; wheat, oats, barley, white rice, milk, butter, ghee, olive, and sunflower oil, any natural sweetener except honey and molasses, sweet fruits (see vata), vegetables (asparagus, pumpkin, cucumber, potato, broccoli, cauliflower, celery, lettuce, zucchini, okra, sweet potato, beans, green beans), coriander, cinnamon, cardamom, fennel, black pepper (in small amounts), chicken, turkey, and egg white.
4. Eat less hot spices, tomatoes, vinegar, alcohol, refined sugar, and acidic or pungent foods (spicy foods, jalapeno peppers, ginger root and cayenne), yogurt, cheese, sour cream, cultured buttermilk, honey, molasses, refined white sugar, some oils (almond, sesame, and corn), some grains (corn, millet, rye, brown rice), grapefruit, sour oranges, sour pineapple, sour plums, papayas, persimmons, olives, radish, beets, onion, garlic, spinach, ginger, cumin, fenugreek, clove, celery seeds, salt, cayenne pepper, mustard seed, cashews, sesame seeds, peanuts, beef, seafood (especially shellfish), and egg yolk.

Overall: Favor sweet, bitter, astringent, cold, heavy, and oily foods, and avoid pungent, sour, salty, hot, light, and dry foods.

KAPHA IMBALANCE TREATMENT

Treat kapha imbalance by teaching clients to (Lansdorf et al., 1993; Collinge, 1996):

1. Choose enjoyable activities and regular exercise.
2. Avoid oversleeping and daytime napping.
3. Arise early to feel lighter and more energetic.
4. Eat more: dry foods, warm foods and drinks, pungent, bitter and astringent foods, of some grains (barley, corn, millet, buckwheat, rye), low-fat milk, honey, apples, pears, pomegranates, cranberries, persimmons, radish, asparagus, eggplant, green leafy vegetables, beets, broccoli, potato, cabbage, carrot, cauliflower, pumpkin, lettuce, celery, sprouts, all spices except salt, all beans except soy, chicken, turkey.

5. Eat less: oily foods; cold or iced foods and drinks; sweet, sour, and salty foods; wheat, rice, or oats; cheese, yogurt, buttermilk, cream, butter; all sweeteners except honey; sweet fruits; tomato, cucumber, sweet potato, zucchini; salt; all nuts; seafood, beef, pork.

In general: Favor pungent, bitter, astringent, light, dry, and hot foods, and eat fewer cold, oily, sweet, sour, salty, or heavy foods.

SCIENTIFIC BASIS

In December 1996, the National Center for Complementary and Alternative Medicine, formerly the Office of Alternative Medicine, released draft reports on pilot studies funded in 1993 and 1994 (OAM, 1996). Three of the studies examined Ayurveda.

One study, conducted by Bala Manyam of the Southern Illinois University School of Medicine, examined the effect of an ayurvedic herb (MPA) derived from the plant Pruriens, in the treatment of Parkinson's Disease. The herb formula was studied for its effect on brain chemicals known to affect Parkinson's. A rat model of anti-Parkinsonism was used. Results showed that the herb was effective in the animal model and contains compounds other than L-dopa that produced the desired effects.

David Simon, of the Sharp Institute for Human Potential and Mind/Body Medicine in San Diego, compared the effects of an Ayurvedic health promotion program with those of a conventional Western health promotion program for ninety enrollees in an HMO. Those in the Ayurveda group followed an Ayurvedic diet, hatha yoga postures, and a regimen of meditation. Those in the Western-style group used progressive relaxation, a conventional Western low-fat, low-salt diet, and brisk walking. A variety of physiological and behavioral outcomes compared the two groups with a third, nonintervention group.

Health-related quality of life improved in both treatment groups, but the Ayurvedic group showed greater improvement. Their scores were statistically higher in general ($p = .04$), for current help perceptions ($p = .01$), and for prescription medication use ($p = .04$).

Yoga was assessed as a treatment for heroin addiction by Howard Schaeffer of the North Charles Institute for the Addictions in Boston. The study examined the effect of weekly yoga in a group setting for clients in an outpatient methadone maintenance program. Effects were compared to traditional group psychotherapy experiences. Composite measures revealed both treatments were equally effective in reducing drug use and criminal activities.

Other research providing evidence of the effectiveness of Ayurveda include the use of the herbal combinations MAK-4 (raw sugar, clarified butter, Indian gallnut, Indian gooseberry, dried catkins, Indian pennywort, honey, nutgrass, white sandalwood, butterfly pea, shoeflower, aloewood, licorice, cardamom, cinnamon, cyperus, and turmeric) and MAK-5 (Gymnema aurentiacum, black musale, heart-leaved moonseed, Sphaerantus indicus, butterfly pea, licorice, Vanda spatulatum, elephant creeper, and Indian wild pepper). These formulas have been shown to be more effective as antioxidants (free radical scavengers) than vitamins C and E (Sharma, Hanna, Kaufman, & Newman, 1992).

Some other studies examined the effect of MAK-5. They also provided evidence of the power of the Ayurvedic approach. A double-blind, placebo-controlled study examined the effects of the herbal combination in 46 individuals with hay fever. The study found significant reductions in allergy symptoms in those taking this herbal combination (Glaser, Robinson, & Wallace, 1991). In the other study, nine individuals took MAK-5 for 3 months. There was a significant decrease in Substance P (a neurotransmitter), suggesting that this herbal formula may help relieve gastrointestinal and pulmonary inflammation and pain without producing toxic effects (Sharma, Hanissian, Rattan, Stern, & Tejwani, 1991).

REFERENCES

Chopra D. (1994). *Perfect Weight: The Complete Mind/Body Program for Achieving and Maintaining Your Ideal Weight.* New York: Crown.

Collinge W. (1996). Ayurveda: The Wisdom of the Ancients. *The American Holistic Health Association Complete Guide to Alternative Medicine.* New York: Warner Books.

Glaser JL, Robinson DK, & Wallace RK. (1991). Improvement in seasonal respiratory allergy with Maharishi Amrit Kalash 5, an Ayurvedic herb immunomodulator. *Proceedings of the American Association of Ayurvedic Medicine* 7(1):6.

Lonsdorf N, Butler V, & Brown M. (1993). *W Woman's Best Medicine: Health, Happiness, and Long Life Through Ayur-Veda.* Los Angeles: Jeremy Tarcher.

OAM. (1996). Pilot studies funded in 1993 and 1994. Http://www.altmed.od.nih.gov.

Sharma H, Hanissian A, Rattan A, Stern S, & Tejwani G. (1991). Effects of Maharishi Amrit Kalash on brain opioid receptors and neuro-peptides. *Journal of Research and Education in Indian Medicine* 10(1):1–8.

Sharma H, Hanna A, Kaufmann E, & Newman H. (1992). Inhibition of human LDL oxidation in vitro by Maharishi Ayur-Veda herbal mixtures. *Pharmacology, Biochemistry and Behavior* 43:1175–1182.

Zucker M. (1995). Women's health: Ayurveda offers ancient solutions for modern times. *Let's Live* (May):61–66.

Zwolski K. (1999). Ayurveda. In C.C. Clark (Ed.), *Encyclopedia of Complementary Health Practices.* New York: Springer Publishing Company.

Zysk K. (1996). Traditional Ayurveda. In M.S. Micozzi (Ed.), *Fundamentals of Complementary and Alternative Medicine.* New York: Churchill Livingston.

13

CHINESE HEALTH AND HEALING

THEORETICAL BASE FOR PRACTICE

In traditional Chinese treatment, humans are viewed as a microcosmic mirror of the universe. Tao (The Way) are the universal principles that operate in the universe and in the human body. Thus, much of the terminology is derived directly from natural phenomena: fire, water, wind, heat, dryness, and dampness. The system is holistic, based on the idea that no single part can be understood except in relation to the whole person. When energies, called qui, in the human system are in dynamic balance, health flourishes. When preventive health fails, and that is a responsibility shared equally by client and practitioner, dis-ease occurs (Reid, 1996).

Modern Western physics has clearly established that matter is nothing more than highly condensed and organized energy. Human energy functions by its dynamic polarity, the principle of yin (moon, midnight, winter, cold, dark, hard, matter, even, female, down below, inside, back, formative, condensing, alkaline) and yang (sun, noon, summer, hot, radiant, soft, energy, odd, male, up, above, outside, front, transformative, expanding, acid).

These two opposite and complementary qualities keep energy moving. They are responsible for balance and they mutually transform each other. Through their transformative union, five elemental energies—Wood, Fire, Earth, Metal, and Water—arise.

These five elements manage the human system functions. In the physical body, they manage body functions and determine the conditions of glands, organs, and tissues. In the energy system or "auric body" they manifest as emotions and feelings. At the mind level, they are related to will, intuition, and creativity.

Each energy generates and increases the one that follows. Deficiencies and imbalances can be supplemented and replenished by using external sources of energy: food, herbs, sunlight, etc. Energy can be cultivated through exercise, massage, herbs, etc. If natural balancing energies fail, physiological illness occurs. For example, an overactive heart (Fire) will overstimulate the spleen (Earth) and serious digestive problems will often occur. The Chinese health and healing practitioner may help rebalance the human system through acupuncture, herbs, or other therapies. Each treatment is a method of energy transfer meant to restore balance (Reid, 1996).

ROLE OF CHINESE PRACTITIONER

In the Chinese system, the practitioner is a guide, advisor, and coach who teaches the client basic ground rules and strategies for optimizing health and wellness. The superior clinician is one who helps clients stay well. Diagnosis is based on observations of the client's physique, characteristic patterns of movement, body secretions, the head and face (hair, eyes, ears, nose, lips, teeth, throat, and facilial skin are closely linked to the internal organs by channels), the tongue, speaking and breathing patterns, and asking the client to talk about complaints/illness.

Table 13.1 shows some diagnoses for the Chinese system.

In the traditional system, the physician visited the home and was paid as long as everyone remained well; once illness befell any member of the family, the practitioner was not paid, and had to pay for the costs of treatment, until health was restored (Reid, 1996). This chapter examines Chinese herbs and nutrition. Consult Chapter 25 for Chinese touch therapies.

Table 13.1 Observations and Diagnoses

Observations	Diagnoses
Red and swollen upper eyelids	Injury to the liver channel by wind-heat
Inflammation of the middle ear or accumulation of excessive earwax	Dampness and heat in the liver and gallbladder
Prolonged thick, foul nasal discharge (indicates an inflammation of the sinuses)	Heat in the gallbladder channel
Trembling in newborns or persistent tics	Stirring of wind in the liver
Red, swollen, and bleeding gums	Upward flaming of stomach heat
Swollen, deep red tongue	Heat in the heart or local infection
Swollen, dark blue-purple tongue	Poisoning
A tongue with teeth imprints along the outer edge	Deficiency symptom-complex of the spleen
Tendency to stick out the tongue or to play with it	Heat in the spleen
Short contracted tongue	Critical disease
Sticky fur on the tongue	Undigested food, infectious disease or illness due to accumulation of phlegm

(continued)

Table 13.1 *(continued)*

Observations	Diagnoses
Curdlike tongue coating	Dyspepsia or retention of phlegm
Peeled coating on the tongue	Vital essence of the stomach is exhausted
Smothering feeling in the chest that is relieved by deep sighing	Stagnation of *qi* due to deep depression of the liver
Dry cough with scanty or thick sticky sputum	Dryness of the lung due to yin deficiency
Headache accompanied by dizziness, ringing in the ears, and pain in the lumbar region	Deficiency symptom-complex of the kidney
Chest pain, accompanied by fever, a suffocating sensation in the chest, and a bitter taste in the mouth	Dampness and heat in the liver and gallbladder
A serious ear ringing that starts suddenly	Fire and wind in the gallbladder channel

Abstracted from Yanchi (1988a), pp. 192–289.

CHINESE HERBS

Chinese herbal treatments have been in continuous safe use for at least five thousand years. They are believed to be safer than allopathic drugs because the active ingredients in herbs are enfolded within the whole plant. Also, herbs are often used in combination. Both these factors tend to buffer side effects. Although Chinese herbs work on a biochemical level, they also function on the energy level. They act by virtue of their natural affinity of *gui jing* (home into meridians) for target organs. They all have flavors (pungent, sweet, sour, bitter, or salty) that work on one of the elemental energies (Metal, Earth, Wood, Fire, or Water). Table 13.2 shows some of the Chinese herbs and herbal combinations used for specific conditions.

Table 13.2   Chinese Herbs and Their Target Organs

Target condition/Organ	Herbs/Herbal formulas
Abcesses	Herba Agrimoniae
Abcesses, tongue	Akebia Quinata
Abortion, threatened	Radix Scutellariae (baikal skullcap root) or Semen Custutae
Addison's disease	Radix Glycyrrhizae (licorice root)
Allergies, generalized	Cyperus 18(SF)

Table 13.2 *(continued)*

Target condition/Organ	Herbs/Herbal formulas
Allergies, sinusitis	Bi Yan Pian
Allergies, food	Lopanthus Anti-Febrile pills (Hsiang Cheng chi Pien)
Angina pectoris	Radix Notoginseng
Anorexia	Herba Agastachis (winkled giant-hyssop)
Appendicitis	Herba Patriniae
Arthritis, rheumatoid	Radix Angelicae Pubescentis
Ascites, due to cirrhosis	Radix Euphorbiae Kansui or Herba Scutellariae Barbatae
Asthma due to wind-cold	Herba Asari (wild ginger) or Radix Glycyrrhizae (licorice root)
Back, weakness	Radix Morindae
Bell's palsy	Jack-in-the-pulpit[a]
Bleeding, nose, stools, uterine	Petiolus Trachycarpi Carbonisatus
Bleeding, lung or stomach	Rhizoma Bletillae
Bleeding, uterine	Herba Schizonepetae
Bleeding, vaginal in pregnancy	Ramulus Loranthi
Blood sugar, high	Yu Mi Xu (Indian Corn)
Boils/carbuncles	Radix Angelicae Dahuricae
Bronchitis	Herba Asari (Wild ginger)
Cancer, breast	Fos Vinca (vinca rosea) or Bulbus Cremastrae (edible tulip bulb) or Taraxacum Officinale (dandelion)
Cancer, cervical	Jack-in-the-pulpit[a]
Cancer, colon	Camptotheca Acuminata (external ointment)
Cancer, esophageal	Fructus et Radix Camptotheca Acuminata (external ointment) or Radix Actinidiae
Cancer, head and neck	Camptotheca Acuminata (external ointment)
Cancer, liver	Herba Scutellariae Barbatae
Cancer, lung	Fructus et Radix Camptotheca Acuminata (external ointment) or Herba Scutellariae Barbatae
Cancer, nasopharnygeal	Bulbus Cremastrae (edible tulip bulb)
Cancer, skin	Rhizoma Zedoariae (external ointment)[b] or Bulbus Cremastrae (edible tulip bulb)

(continued)

Table 13.2   *(continued)*

Target condition/Organ	Herbs/Herbal formulas
Cancer, stomach	Radix Actinidiae or Herba Scutellariae Barbatae
Cancer, urinary bladder	Camptotheca Acuminata (external ointment)
Cancer, uterine cervix	Rhizoma Zedoariae (external ointment)[b] or Bulbus Cremastrae (edible tulip bulb)
Cardiovascular system hypofunction	Radix Ginseng
Cold, common	Radix Angelicae Dahuricae
Cold, common due to cold or wind-heat	Herba Schizonepeta
Colitis, chronic	Dried ginger
Collapse	Dried ginger
Conjunctivitis, chronic	Flos Buddleiae
Constipation	Bitter apricot kernel
Constipation, chronic	Fructus Persica
Convulsions	Radix Gentianae
Convulsions, infant	Concretio Silicea bambusae
Cough, dry	Lo Han Kuo tea
Cough with profuse phlegm	Pinellia Expectorant Pills and Fritillary-Loquat syrup
Cramps, uterine	Corydalis Yan Hu Suo Analgesic
Cystitis, acute	Lung Tan Xie Gan Wan
Cystitis, urinary tract infection	Herba Taraxaci (dandelion herb)
Dermatitis	Radix Sophorae Flavescentis
Diabetes	Radix Ginseng
Diarrhea, chronic	Liu Jun Zi Wan and Wu Ling San
Digestive system in the young and old	Po Chai Pills (Bao Ji Wan)
Dizziness, due to deficiency of liver	White peony root
Drug poisoning	Radix Glycyrrhizae (licorice root)
Exhausted kidney, spleen, and liver (symptoms such as chronic fatigue, tinnitus, high blood pressure, insomnia, male impotence, lower-back pain, frequent urination)	Six Flavor Rehmannia Pills (Liu Wei Di Huang Wan)
Eczema	Radix Arnebiae seu Lithospermi
Edema	Rhizoma Cynanchi Stauntoni
Epilepsy	Jack-in-the-pulpit[a]
Fever, acute	Herba Menthae (peppermint) or Folium Mori (mulberry leaf)

Table 13.2 *(continued)*

Target condition/Organ	Herbs/Herbal formulas
Food poisoning	Huang Lian Su or Radix Glycyrrhizae (licorice root)
Gallstones	Yu Mi Xu (Indian corn)
Headache, with colds or chills	Chuan Xiong Chao Tiao Wan
Headache, with influenza	Herba Asari (wild ginger)
Headache, with hay fever-sinusitis	Bi Yan PIan
Headache, with fever	Yin Chiao Chieh Tu Pien or Zhong Gan Ling
Heart/Liver/Kidneys stimulates endocrine secretions, promotes kidney function, after childbirth tonic, anti-aging, raw herb reduces fevers and inflammations	Rehmannia glutinosa (shou-di-huang)
Heart: cardiac resuscitation	Radix Curcumae
Heatstroke, prevention	Mung bean
Hemorrhaging, postpartum	Folium Nelumbinis
Hemorrhoids, painful	Fargelin High Strength
Hemorrhoids, bleeding	Yunnan Pai Yao
Hepatitis, viral	Radix Glycyrrhizae[c] (licorice root)
Hepatitis, infectious	Radix Isatidis
Hepatitis, chronic	Herba Scutellariae
Hiccups	Cloves
Hypertension	Radix Sophorae Subprostratae Barbatae or Yu Mi Xu (Indian corn)
Hodgkin's disease	Fos Vinca (vinca rosea)
Impotence	Radix Morindae
Impotence, due to hypofunction of kidney	Cloves
Infantile paralysis	Herba Epimedii
Inflammation, skin and perineum	Radix Gentianae
Insomnia, restlessness	Akebia Quinata
Insomnia, with anxiety and fatigue	Healthy Brain Pills
Insomnia, with tension-stress	Schizandra Dream (HC)
Itching, skin	Cortex Dictamni Radicis
Jaundice	Radix Actinidiae
Knees, weakness	Radix Morindae

(continued)

Table 13.2   *(continued)*

Target condition/Organ	Herbs/Herbal formulas
Lactation, insufficient	Akebia Quinata
Laryngitis/loss of voice	Lasiosphaera seu Calvatia
Legs, painful and swollen	Akebia Quinata
Leprosy	Bai Hua She (Viper Snake)[d]
Liver/Kidneys/Heart tonifies liver and kidneys, regulates blood pressure, anti-aging, restores prematurely grey hair, strengthens kidneys and entire lumbar region	Chinese cornbind (ho-shou-wu)
Liver/Kidneys nourishes semen, marrow, cartilage, supports hormone production	Cervus nippon (lu rung)
Liver/Kidneys nourishes bones and cartilage; corrects lumbago due to kidney deficiency, prevents miscarriage, male sexual tonic, reduces hypertension	Eucommia ulmoides (du-jung)
Liver/Kidneys improves night vision, builds strength in legs, calms heart and nervous system, use in stews and soups as a tonic	Chinese wolfberry (gou-ji-dzu)
Lung, failure to expectorate	Rhizoma Cynanchi Stauntoni
Lung, hypofunction	Radix Ginseng
Lung, bloody sputum	Gecko
Lung, tumors and clots	Taraxacum Officinale (Dandelion)
Malaria	Sweet wormwood
Mastitis	Fructus Hordei Germinatus (malt)
Measles	Herba Schizonepetae or Radix Puerariae
Menopause syndromes	Fructus Ziziphi Jujubae (red date)
Menstrual irregularity/excessive flow	Wu Chi Pai Feng Wan (condensed) or Fructus Corni
Mental tension	Cyperus 18 (SF)
Migraine	Corydalis Yan Hu Suo Analgesic
Muscle spasm/tension	Hsiao Yao Wan
Nausea, vomiting	Semen Cardamoni Rotundi (round cardamon seed)
Nephritis	Folium Perillae
Night sweats	Cortex Lycii Radicis or Radix Asparagi (asparagus root)

Table 13.2 *(continued)*

Target condition/Organ	Herbs/Herbal formulas
Numbness of the limbs	Radix Clematidis
Pain, abdominal, pelvic, lumbosacral	Qi Ye Lian
Pain, arthritic	Angelica Pubescens (du huo)
Pain, back or neck	Radix Puerariae
Pain, bone/bone fracture	Rhizoma Drynariae
Pain, heart or pectoral	Fructus Aurantii Immaturus (immature citron)
Pain, joints	Yi Yi Ren (Job's Tears)
Pain, menstrual due to impeded blood flow	Herba Patriniae
Pain, PMS	Hsiao Yao Wan
Pain, rheumatic muscle or joint	Qi Ye Lien Analgesic
Pain, with numbness or nerve pain	AC-Q(HC)[a]
Pain, of internal organs	Corydalis Yan Hu Suo Analgesic
Pain, due to trauma or infection/inflammation	Yunnan Pai Yao
Pain, uterine	Corydalis Yan Hu Suo Analgesic
Paralysis, face and due to strokes	Bai Hua She (Viper Snake)
Pharyngitis	Herba Schizonepetae or Fructus Arctii (Great Burdock achene)
Pneumonia	Herba Houttuyniae
Poisoning, seafood	Gan Jiang (ginger)
Premature ejaculation	Radix Morindae
Prolapsed organs	Radix Bupleuri or Fructus Aurantii Immaturus
Prostatitis	Lung Tan Xie Gan Wan
Prostatitis, chronic	Kai Kit Wan
Psoriasis	Camptotheca Acuminata (external ointment)
Regurgitation, acid	Semen Raphani (radish seed)
Respiratory symptoms of sneezing, runny nose, sore/swollen throat, fever, headache, and stiff neck and shoulders	Honeysuckle and Forsythia
Respiratory and muscular cold symptoms (especially chills)	Common Cold Remedy (Gan Mao Ling) or Fructus Arctii
Snakebite	Herba Scutellariae Barbatae or Dandelion (juice from fresh plants applied to the bite as an antidote)

(continued)

Table 13.2   *(continued)*

Target condition/Organ	Herbs/Herbal formulas
Spasms/cramps, in calves	Mu Gua (Chinese quince)
Spleen/Lung/Kidneys cardiotonic, immune-system booster (especially when undergoing radiation or chemotherapy), regulates blood pressure and blood sugar, improves skin circulation, promotes wound healing	Astragalus (Huang-chi)
Spleen/Liver promotes circulation, sedative, corrects menstrual disorders, controls bleeding, promotes muscular endurance	Angelica (dang-gui)
Spleen/Lung boasts energy, boosts immunity, enhances cerebral circulation, slows aging	Panax ginseng (ren-shen)
Stomach/Intestine, digestive disorders, headaches, dysentery or food poisoning	Curing Pills (Kang Ning Wan)
Stomach, hypofunction	Radix Ginseng
Stones, kidney, gallbladder or bladder	Herba Lysimachiae (loosestrife)
Stools, bloody	Herba Schizonepetae
Stroke, loss of consciousness	Concretio Silicea bambusae
Surgery, injury, sprain, fracture, inflammation, infection, hemorrhage, shock, pain, menstrual pain with excessive bleeding	Yunnan Pai Yao
Swelling	Yu Mi Xu (Indian corn)
Tetanus	Bai Hua She (Viper Snake)[d]
Throat, sore	Herba Menthae or Radix Platycodi
Tonsilitis	Herba Schizonepetae
Toothache	Radix Angelicae Dahuricae
Traumatic bleeding (surgical and otherwise)	Yunnan White Powder (Yunnan Pai Yao)
Tuberculosis	Rhizoma Paridis
Ulcer, peptic	Radix Glycyrrhizae (licorice root)
Ulcers, stomach or lung	Yi Yi Ren (Job's Tears)
Urethritis	Lung Tan Xie Gan Wan
Urethritis, chronic	Passwan
Urination difficulty due to dampness	Water plantain tuber
Urination, frequent due to deficiency in kidney	Gecko

Table 13.2 *(continued)*

Target condition/Organ	Herbs/Herbal formulas
Urination, painful due to pathogenic heat and dampness	Folium Perillae (purple perilla leaf)
Urination, scanty and painful	Akebia Quinata or Yi Yi Ren (Job's Tears)
Urination, scanty and dark	Yi Yi Ren (Job's Tears)
Vaginitis, acute	Yu Dai Wan
Vaginitis, chronic	Chien Chin Chih Tai Wan

[a]Use with care with pregnant women.
[b]Contraindicated with pregnant women.
[c]Incompatible with Radix Euphorbiae Pekinensis, Flos Genkwa, Radix Euphorbiae, and Kan Sui.
[d]Poisonous.

Abstracted from Yanchi (1988b), pp. 49–147; Beinfield and Korngold (1991), pp. 265–321; Reid (1993), pp. 81–159.

THERAPEUTIC FOODS

The six leading causes of death in the United States have all been directly linked to the diet: heart disease, cancer, stroke, diabetes, cirrhosis of the liver, and arteriosclerosis. The Chinese recognized these important links thousands of years ago, which is why diet and nutrition form the first line of defense against disease. Food is thought of as medicine.

Instead of chewing mints for bad breath, swallowing antacids if gas erupts from the stomach or bowels, or gulping milk of magnesia if the bowels are loose, the practitioners using the Chinese healing system search for causes. Rather than masking these signs of poor digestion, the diet is changed (Beinfield & Korngold, 1991).

In the Chinese system, healthy digestion is equivalent to a happy spleen network. The spleen transforms and absorbs food to generate and distribute qi. All activities from the mouth to the large intestine, including the gallbladder, liver, and pancreas, enter into digestion.

Signs of poor digestion include: (1) belching and flatulence, (2) foul taste in the mouth or bad breath, (3) difficult bowel movements and urination, (4) unpleasant odor of urine and feces, (5) discomfort in stomach and intestines, (6) uncontrollable cravings, (7) not feeling satisfied after eating, (8) not knowing what to eat to feel satisfied, (9) any of the following symptoms: headaches, nausea, nasal and sinus congestion, sudden perspiration, skin eruptions, unpleasant hot or cold sensations, or sores in the mouth (Beinfield & Korngold, 1991).

Basic guidelines for use of food as therapy depend on the observable qualities of a food and its experienced effects. *Yams* are excellent for supplementing qi and strengthening *stomach* and *spleen*. They can relieve fatigue and weakness and help build healthy tissue. Cooked *asparagus* has a strong diuretic effect, so it can eliminate heat and dampness, assisting the health of the *kidney* and *heart*. *Eggplant* enriches and moves the blood and benefits the *kidney* and *liver*. *Radishes* are cool and pungent, tending to disperse congestion in the chest, throat, and digestive tract. *Raw celery* and *green pepper* are crisp and sour, moisturizing, cooling, and relaxing the *qi*, thereby assisting the *gallbladder*, *liver*, and *stomach* (Beinfield & Korngold, 1991).

Although it is not always possible to predict the effect of a food on a specific client, sweet foods generally moisturize and supplement *qi*. Too much sweet food creates heat and phlegm. Spicy foods decongest *qi*, but excess of spice can exhaust the *blood*. A sweet food like milk can be soothing if the body is weak and dry, but it can create mucus congestion and inflammation if the body is *hot* and *damp*. Salty foods can supplement *Blood*, but too much can congeal it. Bitter foods empty and clean the body, but too much can dissipate *qi*. Sour foods tone the nerves and viscera, but too much can lead to cramping and pain.

The following dishes are considered medicinal (Reid, 1994):

1. *Chinese wolfberry stew.* Wolfberries are tonic to the liver and kidneys, and may help remedy mild forms of diabetes, improve vision, nourish blood and semen, increase physical endurance, and enhance sexual stamina. Shiitake mushrooms are an ancient Oriental longevity tonic that may enhance immune functions and inhibit cancer cell growth.

2. *Banana fig breakfast shake.* Bananas provide potassium, while molasses is a good source of organic iron (builds hemoglobin) and serves as a mild diuretic. Figs are beneficial to bowel function.

3. *Barley water.* (Barley and water are placed in a pot, brought to a boil, and then strained into a cup.) Barley water is a popular beverage in Japan, Korea, and northern Asia. It serves as a good dietary supplement for bottle-fed infants, decongests the lungs, cools the entire system, is a diuretic, and relieves conditions with excess dampness such as rheumatic complaints. Barley water can be drunk throughout the day, hot or cold. It can be sweetened with a touch of honey, though most individuals drink it plain.

4. *Ginger and scallion-root tea.* This tea is drunk hot as a remedy for flu, colds, and bronchial ailments. It also works well with indigestion, nausea, and seasickness, and is an antidote for seafood poisoning.

5. *Bee pollen and honey.* Bee pollen is a rich source of amino acids, zinc, essential fatty acids, and trace elements. Mixed with honey, it is used as a natural remedy for skin disorders, allergies, and prostate conditions. The drink is often mixed with ginkgo or ginseng extract to give an additional early-morning start.

6. *Hot hibiscus toddy.* Steeping the buds of dried hibiscus flowers with raw sugar or honey provides a hot drink that is cooling to the body. Hibiscus has an affinity for the sexual organs, helping men retain semen and relieve urinary tract discomfort. It relieves PMS and other menstrual disorders in women. It may also help control diarrhea.

7. *Ginseng chicken.* This food is tonic, and is often prescribed for women recovering from childbirth, or for men or women recovering from prolonged illness. It is also used as an anti-aging dish for the elderly. In the healthy, it promotes health, stimulates energy, boosts immunity, and promotes hormone production. When Panax notoginseng (san-chee) is added to the dish, it enhances blood circulation, promotes healing of wounds, and tones the heart.

REFERENCES

Beinfield H, & Korngold E. (1991). *Between Heaven and Earth, A Guide to Chinese Medicine.* New York: Ballantine Books.

Reid D. (1993). *Chinese Herbal Medicine.* Boston: Shambhala Publications.

Reid D. (1994). *The Complete Book of Chinese Health and Healing.* Boston, MA: Shambhala Publications.

Reid D. (1996). *The Shamblhala Guide to Traditional Chinese Medicine.* Boston, MA: Shambhala Publications.

Yanchi L. (1988a). *The Essential Book of Traditional Chinese Medicine. Volume I, Theory.* New York: Columbia University Press.

Yanchi L. (1988b). *The Essential Book of Traditional Chinese Medicine. Volume II, Clinical Practice.* New York: Columbia University Press.

14

FENG SHUI

Feng Shui is the Chinese art of placement. It is based on the theory that clients experience healthier, happier, and more prosperous lives when their home and work environments are harmonious. An auspicious site is one with a harmonious flow of chi, allowing energy to flow in a manner that supports health. Buildings are viewed as dynamic and alive with chi, with the potential to nurture human beings (Collins, 1996).

Likewise, items that are imbued with joyful or happy memories carry positive chi that is capable of sustaining and healing. Items associated with unhappy or upsetting memories do not carry chi and according to the theory, should be discarded.

YIN OR YANG ROOMS

In Feng Shui, there is a conscious striving to balance yin and yang properties. Yin rooms are cavelike, dark, and dim with dark furniture, dim lighting and a low ceiling. Yang rooms are large and sunny, with spare angular furniture. To balance a yin room, brighter lights and warm pastel yang colors are added. To balance a yang room, dark rich colors, soft upholstered furniture, and rounded window treatments are added (Collins, 1996).

THE FIVE ELEMENTS

Five elements—Wood, Fire, Earth, Metal, and Water—are born out of the interplay between yin and yang. Table 14.1 provides information about the five elements.

The five elements nurture and feed each other: Wood feeds Fire, Fire makes Earth, Earth creates Metal, Metal holds Water, Water nurtures Wood. When all five elements are available in an environment, a healthy balance is maintained (Collins, 1996).

The five elements also control each other, thereby achieving harmony: Metal cuts Wood, Fire melts Metal, Water extinguishes Fire, Earth dams Water, and Wood consumes Earth (Collins, 1996).

Table 14.1   The Five Elements

Element	Where found
Wood	All wooden materials
	Plants and flowers, alive and artificial
	Plant-based cloth and textiles (cotton, rayon, etc.)
	Floral prints
	Columnar shapes (like the trunk of a tree)
	Green and blue colors
	Art depicting plants, flowers, gardens, and landscapes
Fire	Pets and wildlife
	Items made from animals: fur, bone, leather, feathers, and wool
	Triangles, pyramids, and cones
	All forms of lighting: electric, oil, candles, natural
	Art depicting people, animals, light, or fire
	All red colors
Earth	Items made from earth: adobe, brick, tile, ceramic or earthenware
	Squares, rectangles, and long flat surfaces
	Art depicting landscapes: desert, fields, earth
	Yellows and earth-tones
Metal	All metals: brass, iron, silver, aluminum, gold, copper, stainless steel
	Circles, ovals, and arches
	Rocks and stones: marble, granite, flagstone, sandstone, etc.
	Crystals and gemstones
	Art and sculpture made from stone or metal
	All whites and light pastels
Water	All water: fountains, streams, rivers, oceans, etc.
	Flowing, free-form, and asymmetrical shapes
	Reflective surfaces: mirrors, glass, cut crystal
	All blacks, blues, and grays

To find the primary path of chi in a building, stand at the door and look through to a window. There should be a meandering, friendly flow. When doors or windows are located directly across from other doors or windows, the chi may flow too quickly to nourish and support. A screen, furniture, plants, or art can slow the flow of chi, making the environment more healthy.

Electrical equipment can activate chi. Anything from a computer to a copier can draw attention to itself and away from the human beings in the environment. This is useful in a work area, but in a sleeping or rest area, electrical equipment can continually call for attention. The best solution is to conceal equipment in a cabinet or cover it with a beautiful cloth.

The Bagua map is used to create powerful changes in clients' lives. Bagua describes the eight basic building blocks of the I Ching. Standing at the front entrance of a building or room, the Bagua, divide the structure into nine equal blocks. The middle left square is the Health and Family square. Wood dominates, together with blues and greens. Knowledge and self-cultivation appears in the front left block (Collins, 1996).

CASE STUDY: *The Health and Family Bagua*

Mr. S. was recuperating from bypass surgery, but spent most of his time in bed. He complained of feeling lethargic and lacked energy to do much of anything. The practitioner explained that the middle left square of his house was his Health and Family area. She asked Mr. S. to picture what was in that room. When he described a dark room with the cat's litter box in it, the practitioner had some ideas. "I suggest you move the litter box to a room on the middle right side and bring in a lamp and wooden table to the health and family room." After talking for a while, the practitioner also suggested Mr. S. leave the door open to that dark room, leave the lamp on at all times to remind him he was healing, place some fresh flowers on the table to symbolize enhanced health, and place a photo of a loved one next to the flowers to convey family love. To stimulate the flow of chi in the room, Mr. S. was asked to hang a mirror framed in wood over the table and a piece of art on the wall that he associated with vibrant health and that contained the colors of all five elements. Finally, the practitioner asked that Mr. S. bring a healthy plant into the health and family room.

On Mr. S's next visit, the client reported that his health had begun to improve and his lethargy disappear as he began to incorporate feng shui principles by changing the dark room. The practitioner theorized Mr. S. was no longer being affected by stagnant dark chi. Instead, he had been nourished by the personal things placed in the Health and Family area that helped his immune system and body recuperative powers to function at a higher level.

FENG SHUI AFFIRMATIONS

Feng Shui also includes displaying affirmations (see Chapter 15) in the Health and Family area. Some affirmations to use are:

- My health is excellent in every way
- I am vibrantly healthy and happy
- Relationships with my family are satisfying
- I enjoy joyful relationships with friends
- I am blessed with loving relationships

GENERAL FENG SHUI INTERVENTIONS

General feng shui interventions can be used in all cases, despite the client problem (Collins, 1996; Govert, 1993).

1. Give away unloved items and fill Bagua areas with possessions that nourish and calm.

2. Close bathroom drains and toilets to keep Chi from flowing out.

3. Make sure the chi flows neither too slow nor too fast in the Health and Family area of the home. Mirrors can be used to stimulate and circulate chi. When doors and windows are opposite each other, when a neighbor's window intrudes into private areas, when two walls in the same room are different heights, when corners protrude, or stairways come careening down from an upper level, mirrors can reflect structural culprits and circulate the chi back around. Mirror tiles, foggy antique mirrors, mirrors hung at heights that cut off images, mirrors hung opposite each other or facing a bed should be avoided because they deplete chi. Hang mirrors across from doors that open onto a hall to widen a narrow hallway and adjust the chi of individuals who enter the hall from a doorway. If a work desk does not face the door, hang a mirror behind it to alert the worker that others are approaching before they arrive.

4. Use lighting to bring additional chi into an area. Lights that point up can symbolically lift a low ceiling. Lampposts or uplighting can anchor a missing Bagua area or symbolically lift a low-lying property. Fluorescent lighting flickers and depletes chi while full-spectrum bulbs, incandescent, and halogen lighting help balance and enhance a Bagua area. To balance a too-large fireplace that threatens to burn up the chi in an area, place a symbol of Water nearby (bowl of water, glass fireplace doors, crystal ornamentation, or an interior water feature); or place healthy plants, fresh flowers, or an artful screen in front of a fireplace not in use.

5. Hang a round faceted crystal, the size of a quarter to a 50-cent piece to balance chi that's moving too fast or slow for comfort or areas dominated by the Fire of a very sunny window. Cut-glass crystal raindrops, heart or octagons can enhance chi when placed near windows to catch the sun in a rainbow.

6. Use windchimes, wind sculptures, bells, and musical instruments to invite in chi. Hang uplifted bamboo flutes to direct chi and play recorded nature sounds that evoke the ocean, a forest, or a meadow to add chi to a stressful environment.

7. Choose healthy plants and fresh flowers to carry chi into Bagua areas. Avoid plants with threatening or sharp or pointed leaves. Artificial plants and flowers may be a better choice when maintenance is a problem; they bring more chi than unhealthy or unkempt living plants. Remove any sickly or dying plants from all Bagua areas and replace them with healthy substitutes. Pets enhance chi and so do birdfeeders.

8. Collect objects of nature—rocks, dried flowers, driftwood, potpourri, shells, pine cones, seed pods, logs and incense—and place them about the house to enhance chi.

9. Place fountains and waterfalls in strategic places to refresh Chi. Use any combination of urns, pools, bowls, and birdbaths filled with clean water to enhance chi.

10. Hang Banners, flags, weathervanes, whirligigs, and mobiles to lift the chi.

11. Use paintings, sculptures, collages, and textiles to enhance chi.

12. Make sure all five elements are represented in every room.

13.   Place an item that symbolizes vibrant health in the Health and Family area.

14.   Use some or all of the following items to enhance the Health and Family area: posters; paintings; collages; photos; figures of ideal health, family and friends, plants and flowers, gardens and landscapes; blue and green items; anything made of wood, including decorations and furniture; momentos, athletic awards, heirlooms or anything that is reminiscent of health and family; floral prints (wallpaper, upholstery, or linens); quotes, affirmations or sayings pertaining to the ideal Health and Family.

REFERENCES

Collins TK. (1996). *The Western Guide to Feng Shui.* Carlsbad, CA: Hay House.
Govert J. (1993). *Feng Shui, Art and Harmony of Place.* Phoenix, AZ: Daikakuji Publications.

C

Mind/Body Approaches

15

AFFIRMATIONS

Accumulating psychoneuroimmunology research provides evidence that the immune system and the central nervous system function as an integrated whole. Thoughts, perceptions, and feelings can alter immunity through two mind-body pathways of communication: autonomic and neuroendocrine. This two-way system confirms that perception affects illness and illness affects perception (Watkins, 1995). It follows that negative feelings and thoughts can affect, if not help create, illness.

Many people use negative self-talk to berate, belittle, produce fear, anger, and other negative feelings that can affect their health status. Mental thought patterns believed to be most detrimental are criticism, anger, and resentment, while love, peace, and joy are believed to be their antidotes (Hay, 1994).

An *affirmation* is a specifically chosen idea that is thought, written, or said, and immersed in consciousness to enhance health (Hay, 1994). Affirmations provide a positive counter-balance for negative self-talk, replacing old patterns of mental thought that can interfere with life satisfaction and optimum health.

Many clients have never received positive reinforcement for changing their behavior. That is why it is important to give praise, affirmative head nods, and smiles as needed to reinforce client attempts at changing. Affirmations are one way clients can give themselves positive reinforcement.

An experiment (Hay, 1994) for both clients and practitioners is to begin every sentence for a week with the phrase, "I love myself therefore . . . " This exercise reveals how unloving and uncaring we are to ourselves, providing an opportunity for changing the way we think about ourselves. It is difficult to begin a sentence with "I love myself therefore" and end with "I will continue smoking" (eating junk food, resenting my brother, etc.).

SCIENTIFIC BASIS

Chakalis and Lowe (1992) examined the affect of subliminal affirmations on short-term memory. Sixty volunteers took a face-name-occupation memory test before and after a 15-minute intervention. They were randomly assigned to one of three groups: no treatment, relaxing music, and subliminal presentation of memory-improvement affirmations embedded in relaxing music. Only the affirmations group significantly improved their performance on recall of names.

CASE STUDY: *Affirmations*

Joanna R., a complementary practitioner, met with Ben H., a client who had been diagnosed with diabetes 5 years ago but who was not following the prescribed meal plan or exercising. As a result his blood sugar had soared and he had gained weight. The practitioner asked Ben if he wanted to try using affirmations. Ben agreed. Together, they phrased the following affirmation: "I, Ben, am finding it easier and easier to follow a vegetarian food plan."

The practitioner asked Ben to say the affirmation aloud and listen carefully to the words. He frowned while saying the words and the practitioner asked him, "How do you feel when you hear yourself saying the words?" "I don't believe it," he said, looking away. The practitioner asked him to repeat the affirmation and report on his feelings. By the time he repeated the affirmation for the fourth time, he smiled and said, "You know, my wife got a new vegetarian recipe book. Maybe we could try some of them."

The practitioner wrote down the affirmation on a 3 × 5 card. The client agreed to carry it with him and tape a copy of it to his dashboard, and put another copy on the freezer section where his wife kept her ice cream. The next visit, Ben told the practitioner he totally agreed with the affirmation and was ready to discuss ways to stick to a vegetarian eating plan.

GUIDELINE FOR USING AFFIRMATIONS

1.　Provide a relaxing, sharing atmosphere. Present affirmations as a new method found useful by many clients with many different kinds of health problems. Ask for full participation in working with you to develop useful affirmations. If the client appears tense or anxious, consider using a relaxation tape prior to developing affirmations.

2.　Obtain information from clients about health issues of current concern. Consider using Table 6.1, Assessment/Treatment/Evaluation, at an initial session to gather data.

3.　Dialogue with clients about the best way to state the affirmation. Affirmations can be stated in contemplation or action modes. Ask clients, "Are you ready to start thinking about changing or are you ready to use affirmations to take action to change?" Sometimes clients may be unsure themselves and think they want to change, but may find during the initial affirmation process that they are not yet ready to change. These clients are really at the contemplation of change stage. Affirmations are useful at either stage, but should be stated in appropriate form: "It's getting easier and easier to smoke 10 cigarettes a day" (behavior mode) vs. "It's getting easier and easier to think about smoking 10 cigarettes a day" (contemplative mode).

4.　Assist clients to state the affirmation in their own words. Actively listen to clients until it is clear how an affirmation might be stated, but then keep checking with clients until they agree the affirmation sounds right for them. For example, "It sounds as if an affirmation for you might be, 'It's getting easier and easier to let go of my angry feelings toward Cora.' How does that sound to you?" Be sure to listen carefully, giving the client time to reflect on your question and answer honestly. Affirmations are best stated in the becoming mode, e.g., "It's getting easier and easier to . . . " or, "I'm becoming more comfortable with the idea of . . . "

5.   Once an affirmation has been agreed upon, write it on a 3 × 5 card, and ask clients to write or say the affirmation 20 times a day, each time listening for an inner response to hearing it said or writing it. Practice this process at least 3 times with the client, asking them, "What is your reaction to hearing yourself say that (read what you've written down)?" After hearing their reaction, ask them to say or write the affirmation again, then ask, "How does it sound this time?" At first, clients may respond with "I'll never be able to do it," or, "I don't believe it." With repetition, their inner responses begin to move toward, "Maybe I can do it."

6.   Advise clients to carry their chosen affirmation(s) with them on 3 × 5 cards and place them in prominent places where they'll be read frequently: briefcase, purse, car dashboard, refrigerator, bathroom mirror, desk, etc. Suggest to clients that hearing themselves say the affirmation, writing it down, and reading it aloud provides additional feedback and thus is potentially more powerful than simply saying or reading it back. Stress the importance of trying out all methods and choosing the best one(s) for that client.

7.   Provide, or have clients provide, an ongoing method of reinforcement for continuing the affirmation.

8.   At the next visit, be sure to check with each client to find out how the process went, if there were any difficulties, and be sure to reward and praise any successes.

9.   Provide support if clients show frustration, lack skills, or expect too much of themselves, e.g., "This is difficult, but you will get it with practice," or "Keep trying, you're making progress," or "Don't expect to change patterns overnight that you've taken years to develop."

AFFIRMATIONS: SHORTCUTS

If time does not allow for helping the client through the process of affirmation-development, develop a positive affirmational statement in the becoming mode, write it on a 3 × 5 card, and hand it to the client. Suggest, "Here is an affirmation you can use to enhance your other treatment. You can change the wording, but keep it positive. Tape copies to your bathroom mirror, refrigerator, dashboard, desk, and wherever else you might read it often. It will help move you toward health."

SOME POSSIBLE AFFIRMATIONS

1.   It's getting easier and easier to stop smoking (follow my food plan, exercise every day, let go of my angry feelings toward my wife, give myself

unconditional love, open my mind to new ideas, relax and let life flow through me, accept change, share my feelings with others, forgive everyone, move forward in life, allow myself to have fun, fall into a deep sleep and awake refreshed, start menstruating regularly and with comfort, learn to be alone and use my time pleasurably, learn to slow my pulse, breathe easily, live pain-free, etc.).

2. I am becoming more relaxed (confident about my job, able to lubricate my vagina at will, control my urine flow, digest my food easily, able to communicate well with my children, comfortable with whatever people say, etc.).

AFFIRMATIONS FOR PARTICULAR CONDITIONS

Table 15.1 provides affirmations for some conditions. Practitioners can develop specific affirmations in concert with each client.

Table 15.1   Affirmations for Specific Conditions

Condition	Affirmation
AIDS	"My immune system is becoming more powerful every moment."
Allergies	"My world is becoming safer and more friendly."
Anxiety/Panic	"I am becoming peaceful and at ease."
Arthritis	"It's getting easier and easier to be free and let others be free."
Asthma	"I am becoming more and more in charge of my life."
Back Pain	"I am learning to trust and accept all support available to me."
Balance/Falls	"It's getting easier and easier to handle everything in my life."
Bladder infection	"It's easier and easier to let go of old ideas and open myself to change."
Bronchitis	"I am learning to stay peaceful and calm."
Bursitis	"It's getting easier and easier to release all anger and live in peace."
Cancer	"It's getting easier and easier to release old secrets, dissolve all hurts, and live in joy."
Cholesterol	"I am learning to clear the channels of my body."
Chronic fatigue	"It's getting easier and easier to feel full of energy and life."
Cough	"My throat is clearing and healing."
Ears	"I listen with loving regard and hear only the good."
Eczema	"My skin is clearing and I feel secure in my life."
Edema	"It's getting easier and easier to release the past."
Feet	"It's getting easier and easier to move forward in my life."
Gall stones	"I joyously release all negative thoughts."
Glaucoma	"I see everything clearly with peace and love."

Table 15.1 *(continued)*

Grief	"I let go fully, remembering the best of all relationships."
Gum disease	"I move decisively through life."
Hay Fever	"I let go of all hurt feelings, all tension, all uncertainty and fear, and breathe in peace, love, and joy."
Heart conditions	"I release all worries and fill myself up with joy, love, and peace."
Herpes	"I allow nothing to irritate me and feel peaceful and in harmony with my surroundings."
Hypertension	"I release the past and live in joy and peace."
Immune disorders	"My body and mind are empowered and free."
Incontinence	"I am in total control of my body."
Indigestion	"I assimilate my food calmly and joyfully."
Infection	"I remain peaceful, allowing nothing to irritate me."
Insomnia	"I slip into restful sleep, releasing all decisions and worries to a greater power."
Irritable Bowel Syndrome	"I relax into life and surround myself with loving kindness."
Kidney/Stones	"I see the good in everything and relax into knowing there is a grand plan."
Laryngitis	"I speak freely and joyfully."
Liver	"I open myself to love."
Memory	"I relax and remember."
Menopause	"I accept and bless my body with loving care."
Multiple Sclerosis	"I let go and flow with the joy of living."
Overweight	"I fill myself up with love and joy, accepting me as I am."
Pain	"I let go of all negativity and let peace and contentment flow through me."
PMS	"I accept my womanly processes, knowing all is well with me."
Pneumonia	"I breathe in peace, love, and joy."
Prostate	"I accept my manly processes, empowering my sexual pleasure."
Respiratory Disorders	"I breathe in life, peace, and joy."
Shingles	"I relax, knowing all decisions are perfect."
Sinus Congestion	"I refuse to allow anyone to irritate me and breathe in peace and love."
Skin Disorders	"I breathe in emotional security, knowing my uniqueness brings positive attention."
Stroke	"My life is joyful and free."
Substance Abuse	"I allow my body to bring me pleasure and joy."

(continued)

Table 15.1   *(continued)*

Throat	"I express my thoughts and feelings calmly with joy."
Tonsilitis	"I release all negatives and breathe in only positives."
Teeth	"I love my decisions, resting securely in their outcomes."
Vaginal Disorders	"I release all sense of loss and honor the beauty of my body."
Varicose Veins	"I work and move forward with positivity, self-confidence, and joy."
Warts	"My body, mind, and spirit are beautiful."

REFERENCES

Chakalis E, & Lowe G. (1992). Positive effects of subliminal stimulation on memory. *Perceptual Motor Skills* 74(3 Pt 1):956–958.

Hay L. (1994). *Heal Your Body*. Santa Monica, CA: Hay Publishing Co.

Ray S. (1976). *I Deserve Love*. Millbreae, CA: Les Femmes.

Watkins AD. (1995). Perceptions emotions and immunity: An integrated homeostatic network. *Q J Med* 88:283–294.

16

ASSERTIVENESS SKILLS

Interacting with other people can be a considerable source of stress (Davis et al., 1995). People who are unable to express their thoughts and feelings directly or who feel unappreciated or exploited often report having psychosomatic complaints such as headaches or digestive problems. *Assertiveness* assists clients to stand up for their legitimate rights without bullying others or being bullied. Being assertive can also lead to feelings of self-confidence, reduced anxiety, decreased bodily complaints, and improved communication with others (Clark, 1996).

Being assertive means clearly taking responsibility for what is expected from others by using I-messages: "I suggest . . . ", "I feel angry . . . ", "I suggest we settle this by . . . "

Aggressiveness has an element of control or manipulation. Often, You-messages are used: "Why didn't you? . . . ", "You should have . . . " Avoidance of issues can quickly build to a blow-up (aggressiveness), blaming the other person(s) and refusing to take responsibility for feelings. This blow-up is often followed by a period of guilt, and the pattern recurs, shifting next to a build up of resentment (Clark, 1996).

Assertiveness skills can break this destructive pattern by offering a way to clear communication of feelings and expectations and a reduction in blow-ups and guilt.

Clients can be taught a number of different strategies to enhance their assertiveness and reduce their stress including relaxation exercises (see chapter 23) and feedback practice. There are a number of strategies to use to provide feedback about assertive presentation of self. Mirror practice gives feedback about facial expression, posture, and fit of words with gestures and body position. It can also be helpful as a rehearsal for assertive statements prior to the real-life situation.

Audio- and videotape recorders also provide practice in assertiveness, including clues about whether there are sufficient pauses, assertive tone and pace, firm quality, and whether the issue is clearly stated and adhered to. The content of tape practice can provide valuable information about the ability to limit interruptions, express feelings appropriately, take a stand on an issue, disagree, admit a mistake, reward or thank another person, give positive criticism, say no, express distress about a relationship, and ask for collaboration (Clark, 1996).

Another use of audiotape is to record relaxing or rewarding messages that can be played at a later time. Videotape feedback adds information about eye contact, body posture and positioning, gestures, facial expressions, directness of verbal response, conciseness, and confidence of presentation. Videotape scripts can be written and then recorded and evaluated.

Another way to use videotape is to record role playing upcoming situations that have been identified by the client as potentially difficult. Clients can role play these situations with practitioners or with family or friends and tape their conversations. Afterward, clients can review the tapes and evaluate their performance. They can try the role playing situation again, modifying what they say and how they say it until they feel satisfied.

SPECIFIC USES OF ASSERTIVENESS SKILLS

Assertiveness skills can be used to reduce anger, depression, anxiety, antisocial aggressive behavior, marital discord, low self-esteem, team skills, and other work-related behaviors.

The skill can be modeled or clients can be shown a brief videotape that exemplifies the assertive skill needed. The entire verbal and nonverbal behaviors are then imitated by the client. New behaviors are established and avoidant behaviors reduced by this method. A group setting is very effective. Clients can work in pairs practicing assertive responses, then videotape the scene, and view and repractice until they are pleased with their performance.

A client's behavior may need to be prompted or "shaped" with comments such as, "Look me right in the eye when you say that," or "Speak a little louder and more firmly," or "Tell me you won't be able to work overtime tonight, but will try to help out next week." Practicing new behaviors in the safety of the practitioner's office reduces discomfort. Sometimes 5 or 10 minutes of practice is sufficient for a simple assertive encounter.

Covert modeling is as effective as actual rehearsal (Kazdin, 1975). So, if office time is short, have clients view a video of assertive behavior, then send them home with the homework assignment of picturing themselves dealing effectively with the situation. If the practitioner has not attended an assertiveness class, it would be wise to do so prior to teaching clients to be assertive. Not only will assertiveness skills be current, but handouts and resource materials will be available to pass on to clients.

Anger Reduction

Social skills training programs are based on the theory that angry people become embroiled in aggressive encounters because they have not developed alternative, adaptive behaviors (Fodor, 1992). An anger reduction program includes asking clients to:

1. Identify what makes you angry and under what circumstances.
2. Use relaxation techniques to cope with emotional arousal (see Chapter 23 for directions).
3. Simulate anger-provoking situations. Use self-talk to stay calm: "I don't need to prove myself. This is a small thing and I can handle it." "Take a deep breath and take each issue point-by-point." "Don't take this personally." "I could have gotten more upset, but I stayed pretty calm."
4. Repeat anger-stimulating situations and calming self-talk until client feels capable of managing anger.

Depression

Lack of social skills, at least in adolescents, is highly correlated with depression (Fodor, 1992). Depressed individuals often isolate themselves from peers by displaying no verbal or nonverbal behaviors that would invite peer interaction. Some of the practice behaviors needed include: maintaining eye contact with others, initiating a conversation, taking turns talking with a partner, and identifying what they did well as well as what they need to work on when talking to others.

A homework form for clients with depression might resemble Table 16.1 below. Clients can be asked to videotape their practice sessions and then self-assess themselves on the behaviors, ranking themselves from 1 to 5 by circling where they stand, and starring those behaviors they want to work on.

Substance Abuse

A crucial skill for substance abusers is the ability to say no. Substance abusers have low self-esteem and negative self-image. Abstaining from drugs and/or alcohol brings about a mourning process expressed by denial, anger, self-pity,

Table 16.1 Practice Behaviors for Reducing Depression

Behaviors	Assessment				
	Needs work				Excellent
Making eye contact	1	2	3	4	5
Initiating a conversation	1	2	3	4	5
Taking turns talking	1	2	3	4	5
Clear and concise words	1	2	3	4	5
Sticking to the issue	1	2	3	4	5
Using "I" statements	1	2	3	4	5
Tone of voice	1	2	3	4	5
Speed of talking	1	2	3	4	5

depression, and finally acceptance. Many are consumed by self-hate for the problems they have caused. Pressures can mount when they try to live without drugs or alcohol, and without the proper tools, relapse is likely (Fodor, 1992).

Clients who abuse substances can use the following behaviors to help them stay away from drugs or alcohol:

1.   Practice relaxation exercises to reduce anxiety so they can live without drugs or alcohol.

2.   Avoid persons, places, and things that might influence them to use again.

3.   Use self-statements to maximize refraining from using psychoactive substances, including: "No, it isn't worth it.", "No, I won't do it.", "No way will I throw away what I've been working for."

4.   Practice self-affirming statements to use when others challenge their ability, e.g., "I'm a different person now; I'm capable of handling the job (school, relationship).", "I have not relapsed and I'm not going to.", "I deserve to try to enter a college of my choice, not one someone else picked out for me."

REFERENCES

Clark CC. (1996). *Wellness Practitioner: Concepts, Research, and Strategies.* New York: Springer Publishing Company.

Davis M, Eshelman ER, & McKay M. (1995). *The Relaxation and Stress Reduction Workbook.* Oakland, CA: New Harbinger Publications.

Fodor I. (1992). *Adolescent Assertiveness and Social Skills Training, A Clinical Handbook.* New York: Springer Publishing Company.

Kazdin AE. (1975). Covert modeling, imagery assessment and assertive behavior. *Journal of Consulting and Clinical Psychology* 43:716–724.

17

BREATHING

Breathing is important to hand temperature (Bacon & Poppen, 1985), the cardio-vascular system (Cacioppo & Petty, 1982), electro-encephalogram readings (Rampil, 1984), and reaction time (Beh & Nix-James, 1974). Disordered breathing can affect the endocrine, cardiovascular, and nervous systems because it creates an acid-base imbalance. Breathing rate also affects blood pressure, heart rate, respiratory sinus arrhythmia, and stroke volume. Hyperventilation should be considered in cases of mitral prolapse, anxiety states, panic attacks, phobias, burnout and posttraumatic stress disorder, angina pectoris, myocardial ischemia and infarction (Fried & Grimaldi, 1993).

Health and wellness can be enhanced by numerous breathing methods. Several are discussed. Prior to using any breathing method, an assessment is suggested.

BREATHING ASSESSMENT

When clients first enter the office, there are numerous observations that can be made to assess breathing. Table 17.1 provides an assessment form to use to assess breathing.

BREATHING EXERCISE CAUTIONS

Ensure there is no condition that contraindicates the use of breathing training. Low blood pressure (blood pressure can plummet) and diabetes (reduces insulin dependence) are two conditions that should be red flagged for caution. Some clients experience airway or breathing difficulties when asked to focus on their breathing process (Post-White, 1998). In these cases, another treatment should be used.

As innocuous as the exercises that follow appear, it is wise to use them cautiously as there is the remote possibility that a particular client may have a preexisting condition that makes the exercises hazardous. Always proceed with training slowly, evaluating the response of the client to breathing training. For

Table 17.1   Breathing Assessments

Assessment	Meaning
Shake the client's hand	Warm, cold, moist, or dry hands indicate arousal
Ask: "How do you spell your name," then observe for chest heaving	Air hunger or dyspnea is a sign of chronic hyperventilation
Look to see if clothes are tight at belt level	Restrictive clothes can impede breathing
Obtain client permission, then palpate the neck for tightness/tension	Constricted muscles at neck and throat level can impede smooth breathing
Ask which of the following are ingested: alcoholic beverages, yeast breads or any food made with yeast, breads and crackers containing cheese, sour cream, beef or pork or chicken liver, canned meats, canned meat extracts or gravies, salami or sausage, aged cheese, soy sauce, eggplant, salted dried fish, herring or cod, pickled herring, Italian broad beans, any spoiled or improperly stored food	All of these foods contain tyramine or contain bacteria with enzymes that can convert tyrosine to tyramine; all potentiate blood vessel change and hyperventilation
Ask if the client has any of the following symptoms: tension, fatigue, inability to concentrate, a sense that things are unreal, depression, anxiety, panic attacks, phobias/fears, dyspnea, tachypnea, air hunger, headaches, migraine, Raynaud's syndrome, gastritis, indigestion, chest pain, stress (family and other coping problems), impaired immune system (frequent colds, tonsilitis, or ear infections), frequent allergy symptoms, bronchitis, or chronic vaginal yeast infections	These are the symptoms most apt to be encountered in clients with hyperventilation syndrome

Sources: Abstracted from Fried & Grimaldi, 1993; Garrison & Somer, 1995.

clients unused to deep abdominal breathing, they may find the exercises strenuous. Tell these clients: "Tell me right away if you experience any discomfort." If a client looks distressed or complains of discomfort, stop the exercise immediately.

DIAPHRAGMATIC AND ALTERNATE NOSTRIL BREATHING METHODS

Many breathing exercises use abdominal or nose breathing to achieve positive effects. This section examines two types of diaphragmatic breathing and alternate nostril breathing. In all cases, give the client an explanation for using the exercise, e.g., "Now you will be doing a breathing exercise that has been very useful for getting people to relax, reduce muscle tension, and feel more peaceful. Start slowly and let your breath flow effortlessly, making sure you feel comfortable at all times. Be sure to keep your mouth closed and breathe only through your nose."

Trainees may experience breathing difficulty as the inability to get enough air. Once they see that changing their breathing patterns results in effortless diaphragmatic breathing, they can relax and allow the air to flow in (Fried & Grimaldi, 1993).

Diaphragmatic Breathing

Diaphragmatic respiration is the voluntary control of abdominal breathing. It is superior to shallow or chest breathing (Hughes, 1979). There are several ways to teach clients diaphragmatic breathing.

First Diaphragmatic Breathing Method.   Directions to give clients include:

1. Lie down with bent knees supported by pillows, and your hands resting on your lower front ribs.
2. Pay attention to the upper rib movement until your breathing quiets.
3. Pay attention to abdominal movements until the abdomen relaxes and distends on inspiration.
4. Make your exhale twice as long as your inspiration until it lasts for 10 to 15 seconds without loss of control of the next inhale.
5. Sit up, feet apart and arms relaxed.
6. Lean forward while exhaling, until your head is near or between your knees while firmly contracting abdominal muscles.
7. Slowly uncoil during inhale.
8. Next, lie on your back with your knees drawn up.
9. Draw one knee up to your chin while exhaling and lower it while inhaling.
10. Repeat with the other knee.
11. Repeat with both knees, keeping your shoulders and arms relaxed.
12. Practice maintaining this breathing pattern while sitting or standing.

Second Diaphragmatic Breathing Method.   Another method of diaphragmatic breathing includes giving clients the following directions:

Lie on your back and place your left hand on your rib cage as a guide that limits its movement. Place your right hand on your abdomen over the umbilicus. While inhaling deeply through your nose, make an effort to push your abdomen out and up. If the hand on your abdomen moves when you breathe in, you are doing the exercise correctly. Try to exhale for twice as long as you inhale.

Alternate Nostril Breathing

Alternate nostril breathing consists of directing clients to breathe through the nose. There is a known shift in laterality in nasal breathing. As the tissues in one nostril swell, the tissues in the other recede. About every one and three-quarter hours, this cycle alternates. Physiological and cognitive changes accompany the predominance of left or right nostril breathing (Klein, Pilton, Possner, & Shannahoff-Khalsa, 1986).

Training includes asking the individual to focus on the sensations created by air flowing through the nostrils including:

1. Place your left index finger lightly over your left nostril.
2. Press only hard enough to close it.
3. Inhale through your right nostril.
4. Press your right index finger on your right nostril.
5. Press and exhale through your left nostril.
6. Repeat, inhaling through your left nostril and exhaling through your right while keeping the opposite nostril lightly closed.

Alternate nostril breathing gives the practitioner a chance to observe the client and notice any obstruction, swelling, deviation of the septum, etc. The procedure also demonstrates to the client that it is not easy to hyperventilate when breathing through the nose; this is of great use to clients who hyperventilate when anxious.

ADDITIONAL RECOMMENDATIONS

Whichever breathing exercise is used, it may be helpful to use the following statements: "Please sit back in your chair. Let yourself relax into the chair."

It is also possible to combine guided imagery with breathing, enhancing the relaxation process. The practitioner first determines whether the client likes the beach. If yes, the practitioner can say, "I'm going to give you directions to imagine you are on your favorite beach, comfortable, relaxed. Please close your eyes, or leave them open if that is more comfortable for you. The sun is shining, it feels warm on your shoulders. Let that warmth flow through you . . . and down your shoulders and arms and out your fingertips. The ocean is calm and refreshing."

When the client inhales, say: "The surf is coming in gently." When the client exhales, say, "The surf is going out gently." Continue making these statements as the client breathes and relaxes.

BREATHING EXERCISES FOR SPECIFIC CONDITIONS

Anxiety and Panic

Ask clients who are suffering from extreme anxiety or panic to demonstrate the problems they are having with breathing. After noting the constricted breathing pattern, tell clients that diaphragmatic breathing can help. If they agree, teach clients the following method:

1. "On inhalation, picture air coming up through the feet and legs, filling up the abdominal area, then the chest, exhaling down the arms and out the fingertips."
2. "When you inhale, I'm going to put my hands on your abdomen and sides and ask you to 'bubble out' where I press."
3. (After client has mastered that) "Now I'm going to use the palms of my hands to press down on the tops of both your shoulders." (If that does not work, gently rock or tap the shoulders.)
4. Provide an holistic breathing experience by asking clients to "Talk about what you feel when you let your stomach expand," and "Talk about what you feel letting your shoulders relax."

Asthma

Diaphragmatic breathing may be especially helpful for clients with asthma. They often hold air in reserve, being able to inhale readily, but do not exhale quite as fully as most nonasthma clients. Teaching these individuals to pull back the abdomen with each exhale will improve expiratory volume. This, in turn, enhances inspiratory volume (Fried & Grimaldi, 1993).

Following a baseline recording, ask clients to: (1) pull the stomach in slightly at the end of exhalation, relaxing the shoulders and chest; (2) inhale slowly, letting the tummy "bubble out" completely before filling the chest. It is suggested that the practitioner demonstrate the breath several times, then complete several more breaths with clients. If clients have difficulty focusing on abdominal breathing, ask them to not use their chests at all to breathe. Only when abdominal breathing is well controlled can clients be told to let their chest fill with air at the end of inhalation.

If clients are also seeing an allopathic physician, it is helpful to suggest they share the fact that they are using breathing exercises. It may also be useful to let the allopath know that after some training it may be feasible to reduce the client's medication, under physician supervision.

Cold Extremities

There is a connection between the subjective mind and the vasomotor reflexes. The client needs to learn how to raise local temperature in order to evoke the response. With clients who have cold hands or feet, ask them to focus on breathing warmth into the cold extremity.

Emphysema

Clients with emphysema have a low and flat diaphragm with limited excursion. The chest is relatively fixed during inhaling, resulting in decreased capacity to exhale. As a result, accessory respiratory muscles, namely the scaleni, the pectoralis major, the shoulder girdle muscles, and the sternocleidomastoid muscles are used. Together, they elevate the sternum and the first two ribs to increase inspiratory volume (Johnston & Lee, 1976; Fried & Grimaldi, 1993).

Control of the mechanics of breathing may be minimal at first because clients may have difficulty restraining their chest. To avoid fatigue, they may have to start with 2 to 3 breaths. Clients who have difficulty learning diaphragmatic breathing may need EMG biofeedback to learn the method. Once they use their diaphragm, rather than accessory muscles, inspiratory and expiratory volume increases. Because of the fragility of alveoli in emphysema, clients should be directed not to do breathing exercises at home (Fried & Grimaldi, 1993).

Menopausal Hot Flashes

Training in simple breathing procedures can result in a significant reduction in hot flashes associated with menopause. Breathing exercises are a valid alternative to hormone replacement therapy for hot flash treatment (Freedman & Woodward, 1992).

Migraine

Migraine is a vascular event related to impaired regional cerebral blood flow. Symptoms are reported to be less severe after breathing training (Fried & Grimaldi, 1993).

Panic Disorder

Fried and Grimaldi (1993) maintain that panic attacks and other stress symptoms may be due to hyperventilation, rather than vice versa. This could explain why breathing exercises reduce panic.

REFERENCES

Bacon J, & Poppen R. (1985). A behavioral analysis of diaphragmatic breathing and its effects on peripheral temperature. *Journal of Behavior Therapy and Experimental Psychiatry* 16:15–21.

Beh HC, & Nix-James DR. (1974). The relationship between respiratory phase and reaction time. *Psychophysiology* 11:400–412.

Cacioppo JT, & Petty RE. (1982). *Perspectives in Cardiovascular Psychophysiology.* New York: Guilford Press.

Freedman RR, & Woodward S. (1992). Behavioral treatment of menopausal hot flushes: Evaluation by ambulatory monitoring. *Am J Obstet Gynecol* 17:305–306.

Fried R, & Grimaldi J. (1993). *The Psychology and Physiology of Breathing.* New York: Plenum.

Garrison R, & Somer E. (1995). *The Nutrition Desk Reference.* New Canaan, CT: Keat Publishing.

Hughes RL. (1979). Does abdominal breathing affect regional gas exchange? *Chest* 76:288–293.

Johnston R, & Lee K. (1976). Myofeedback—a new method of teaching breathing exercises in emphysematous patients. *Physical Therapy* 56:826–829.

Klein R, Pilton D, Possner S, & Shannahoff-Khalsa DS. (1986). Hemispheric performance efficiency varies with nasal airflow. *Biological Psychology* 23:127–137.

Post-White J. (1998). Imagery. In M. Snyder & R. Lindquist (Eds.), *Complementary/ Alternative Therapies in Nursing.* New York: Springer Publishing Company.

Rampil IJ. (1984). Fast Fourier transformation of EEG data. *Journal of the American Medical Association* 251:601.

18

COPING SKILLS TRAINING

Coping skills training procedures grew out of relaxation therapy and systematic desensitization procedures that were expanded and refined by Meichenbaum and Cameron (1974). The procedures combine progressive relaxation and coping self-statements that are used to replace defeatist self-talk evoked by stressful situations.

Coping skills procedures are used in rehearsals for real-life events identified as stressful. A stressful situation is called forth, progressive relaxation is practiced, and then coping skills statements are repeated until the situation can be rehearsed without feeling stressed.

The procedures have been shown to be effective in the reduction of general anxiety, and anxiety related to speaking, interviews and tests, and in the treatment of phobias, especially the fear of heights. In a 2-year follow-up study, Davis, Eshelman, and McKay (1995) reported 89% of hypertense, postcardiac clients were able to achieve general relaxation using coping skills, and 79% controlled tension, fall asleep sooner, and slept more deeply. It takes approximately 1 week to master coping skills procedure use once progressive relaxation has been learned.

Coping statements for each stage of a stressful situation follow. Clients can develop their own list and memorize them and/or carry a copy with them.

Preparatory stage

- I can handle this.
- I'll jump right in and be all right.
- Soon this will be over.
- There's nothing to worry about.
- It will get easier and easier once I start.

During the Situation

- Take a deep breath and relax.
- I will not allow this situation to upset me.
- I can do this: I'm doing it now.
- Deep breathing really works.

- I can keep my mind on the task at hand.
- I can take this step by step.
- I'll feel very good when this goes well.
- My fear is leaving me; I can watch it go down as I relax.
- I can keep my body free of tension.
- If I focus on what I have to do, I can crowd out any fears.

Reinforcing Success

- I did well.
- By not thinking about being afraid, I wasn't afraid.
- Situations don't have to overwhelm me any more.
- I'm getting healthier.
- I can turn worry off.
- I'm going to tell _____ (friend or family) about my success.
- I did it!

CASE STUDY

Emily had been afraid of heights since she was 5 years old and someone tried to push her out a window. For many years she controlled her fear by living and working on the ground floor. When she was offered a job with much more responsibility and pay, she had to turn it down because she had to take an outside elevator to the tenth floor and she was afraid she might get dizzy or be unable to step inside the elevator.

She found out about a counselor who used coping skills training and visited him. He taught her relaxation skills and wrote out some coping skills statements for her to use. She practiced riding only to the first floor for a day, then took the elevator up more floors, always practicing the coping skills statements and rewarding her success. By the seventh day, she was able to take the elevator to the tenth floor and felt comfortable doing so.

GUIDELINES FOR INTEGRATING COPING SKILLS INTO PRACTICE

1. Practice teaching the client relaxation skills, including abdominal breathing. They are the cornerstone of coping skills training. Relaxation should be overlearned so it can be automatically called upon when a stressful situation occurs.

2. Ask the client to build a clear picture of the stressful situation while simultaneously noticing any sign of tension in the body or any hint of anxiety.

3. Ask the client to imagine the stressful situation. The first day imaging three or four stressful scenes may be sufficient and will not overly tire out or turn off the client. If the client has difficulty imagining the scene, read the particulars into a tape recorder and ask the client to take it home and listen to it while picturing the scene.

4.   Once the client masters relaxation skills, it is time to create a personal list of stress-coping thoughts. They should be positive and act as tranquilizers for a tense stomach or tight back. Coping statements should be fear-conquering statements that coach the client to be calm and feel confident. Together with the client, choose from the list suggested above or write similar ones that appeal to the client.

5.   Encourage the client to carry the coping skills statements with them on 3 × 5 cards, to tape them on night tables, kitchen sinks, refrigerators, work desks, wherever they may be read.

6.   When the client is ready, the final stage is applying coping skills statements in the real-life situation. Remember to tell the client that some setbacks are expected because it is more difficult to deal with real-life situations because they are more unpredictable and difficult to control.

REFERENCES

Davis M, Eshelman ER, & McKay M. (1995). *The Relaxation and Stress Reduction Workbook.* Oakland, CA: New Harbinger.

Meichenbaum D, & Cameron R. (1974). Modifying what clients say to themselves. In MJ Mahone, CE Thoresen (Eds.), *Self-Control: Power to the Person.* Monterey, CA: Brokks/Cole.

19

EXERCISE/MOVEMENT

ADVANTAGES OF REGULAR EXERCISE/MOVEMENT

Movement is a simple and effective method of reducing stress that practitioners can recommend to their clients. It also lowers cholesterol, moderates appetite, and prevents aging and some chronic conditions, including obesity, joint and spinal disc disease, muscular tension, high blood pressure, colon cancer, breast cancer, depression, anxiety, osteoporosis, fatigue, coronary heart disease, and stroke.

Movement and exercise can reduce joint stiffness, enhance self-image and self-confidence, reduce depression, increase circulation, decrease blood pressure, positively affect work performance, enhance sleep and the ability to relate to others, enhance breathing ability, and decrease the need for stimulants (National Headache Foundation; Shinton & Sagar, 1993; Angotti et al., 1994; Pate, Rate, & Blair, 1995; and The President's Council on Physical Fitness and Sports).

Exercise has been shown to cut the risk of developing noninsulin-dependent diabetes in men (Manson et al., 1992), and breast cancer in women (Henderson et al., 1994). It also extends life for those over age 70 (Rakowski & Mor, 1992), results in fewer health care claims (Bernacki, 1987), and reduced absenteeism and turnover in the workplace (Shephard, 1983).

THE MEANING OF BODY MOVEMENT

When there is a wholeness to the body/mind/spirit, expression of feelings flows easily. Infants are born flexible and with easy movement. When the flow of energy in the body is disrupted, wholeness is disrupted. As individuals grow, experiencing feelings and not expressing them directly results in breaks in the normally smooth curves of the body. Everyone has some breaks. The difference in magnitude and quantity differentiates clients from having energy blocks to enjoying effective movement and easy energy flow (Kurtz & Prestera, 1984).

Feeling can be "locked" in a body part. For example, instead of striking out in anger, individuals may hold their anger in their abdominal area, leading to digestive upsets and a tight, tense abdomen that may be held in excessively. Or, sadness and lack of grieving can result in a tense jaw, chest, stomach, diaphragm, and some throat and facial muscles. When the feeling is allowed its natural outlets, these areas move spontaneously (Kurtz & Prestera, 1984).

Blocks impede the normal flow of energy. Tension in muscles increases, circulation is constricted, and skin tone and temperature change. Rings of held-in feelings can often be observed in the major segments of the body: neck and upper shoulders, the diaphragm, the lower back between the abdomen and pelvis, the groin, the knees and the ankles; feet and eyes can also be held.

Gross changes in function follow chronic holding. The abdomen may be blown up, while the chest is collapsed. Hands and feet may be small and cold. With a muscular tension in these areas, blood supply is reduced and tissue wastes collect, setting up a mechanism for toxic spasm and stasis. The nervous system responds by firing more signals, leading to a pain-spasm-pain-spasm of a headache, backache, or heartache. As time passes, the tissues harden to splint the area from further attack and a structural block appears where originally an emotional block was (Kurtz & Prestera, 1984).

So, a backache may be the product of a slipped disc, but the original insult may be an emotional one that resulted in an attempt to hold oneself up or back. A heart attack can be viewed as the end result of blocked impulses to love or be loved, that became a block in energy flow, a decrease in circulation, a pooling and thickening of blood, and eventually a physiological blockage.

Harmony with gravity aids in reaching up and out in the world. Disharmony leads to attempts by the body to compensate. If the chest is going in and down, the belly may compensate by going out and up. The ideal axis for attaining the best balance for the body is that point connecting points at the top of the head, middle of the shoulder, midpoint of the hip joint, center of the knee joint, and center of the ankle joint (Kurtz & Prestera, 1984).

The way the body is held or moved can express unresolved feelings. Bodies that bend forward express feelings of being overburdened. Bodies bent backward may experience life as an unending struggle. Stiffness in the legs and feet or locked knees may indicate bracing against a fall. Clients with rigid legs have difficulty bending their toes forward or backward (an indicator of the condition). Movement and position of the feet can also provide important information about how reality is dealt with by the way the ground is contacted. When one foot points in one direction and the other points in another direction, it could indicate confusion. Feet rotated outward put added stress on the ankle and knee joints, while feet facing forward reduce stress, allowing more effective weight transfer through the center of the foot.

Limited sexual, anal, and urinary expression can be assessed in clients with knees that are quite separate with a space between the thighs terminating in a high peak in the midline, as well as in clients whose thighs are drawn inward, squeezing the genitals. Chronic contraction of both the buttocks and thighs restricts energy flow.

The position of the pelvis also reveals inner feelings. A tucked pelvis under tight buttocks allows for a dribbling out of emotion. The retracted pelvis is unable to release and remains cocked, ready to fire (Kurtz & Prestera, 1984). Choosing the correct exercise or movement treatment is related to body energy constrictures and level of flexibility.

Some measures of flexibility (thumb, metaphalangeal extension, and foot arch) are determined by heredity and cannot be changed. Other measures can be improved upon through exercise. These include shoulder stretch, thigh stretch, heel cord flexibility, and ability to touch the floor with the fingertips without bending the knees (Marshall, 1981).

ASSESSING BODY ENERGY BLOCKS

Because blocks can lead to constrictions in body function, it may be useful to assess the structural presentation of clients. Table 19.1 provides information for assessing body energy blocks.

FLEXIBILITY ASSESSMENTS

Flexibility, or its lack, provides clues for future injuries or conditions. There are two measures of flexibility: momentary and chronic. Momentary flexibility changes due to the emotion of the moment. Muscles tighten, breathing rises toward the throat, and the body stiffens. Chronic inflexibility develops from years of not using the body appropriately or may be due to accident, surgery, and/or chronic inhibited emotion.

Practitioners can assess flexibility in several ways: observe the body in movement, ask clients what areas of the body "feel" tight or stiff, or ask clients to complete a range of motion or extension exercises. Asking a client to walk away from and then toward the practitioner will reveal aspects of flexibility. Various regions of the body can also be assessed for flexibility.

Thumb Flexibility

Thumb flexibility can be assessed by pushing the tip of the client's nondominant thumb back toward the forearm. An angle more than 70 degrees indicates better than average flexibility; 60–70 degrees is average; and less than 60 degrees indicates less than average flexibility (Marshall, 1981).

Metacarpal-Phalangeal Extension

Metacarpal-phalangeal extension can be assessed by asking clients to lift and hold up an arm with elbow bent. Push the index finger back toward the wrist. According to J. Marshall, a former chief of sports medicine, more than a 115

Table 19.1   Assessing Body Energy Blocks

Ask clients to stand with hands at their sides, feet together. Observe their bodies using the following questions as a guide.

Front View	Pretreatment	Posttreatment

1. Contrast the upper body with the lower body. Do they appear to fit? Is there a mismatch?
2. Contrast the right side of the body with the left side for symmetry. Is one side more developed, more forward, more back?
3. Is the mouth tight or relaxed?
4. Are the eyes the same size and do they show the same amount of openness?
5. Is the head tilted to one side or the other?
6. Are the shoulders level or is one higher than the other?
7. Is one shoulder longer than the other
8. Is the chest hyperextended, concave, relaxed?
9. Are both arms the same distance from the body?
10. Are the hips level or is one hip higher than the other?
11. Is the pubic area pulled in toward the center of the body or is the abdomen flat?
12. Are the knees facing in or out?
13. Are the knees and lower legs relaxed or tense? (Place one hand behind the lower leg and push slightly. If the knee bends easily it is relaxed; if not, assess the degree of tenseness)
14. Do both feet face forward or does one or both face out?
15. Does energy appear trapped? (Especially observe the chest area.)
16. Is the head tilted up, down, or is it level?
17. Are the shoulders tilted forward or back?
18. Are the scapula flat and level on both left and right side?
19. Is the lower back swayed with the abdomen pushed out or is there a small curve in the small of the back?
20. Is the pelvis tipped out or back?
21. Draw an imaginary line through the ear, shoulder, elbow, hip socket, knee, and ankle. Where is the line out of line or unaligned?

Table 19.1   *(continued)*

Back View

22. Observe for areas where energy appears trapped
    (look over- or underdeveloped), especially in the
    upper back and buttocks.

Look back at the assessment and hold your body as the client does, but exaggerate the posture. What current or potential problems might occur to joints, body parts, internal organs, breathing, circulation, digestion, or elimination based on what you have observed? Validate any conclusions with clients. If problems have not surfaced yet, counsel them to take preventive movement and exercise action.

degree angle indicates high flexibility; 105–115 degrees indicates average flexibility, and less than 105 degrees indicates less than average flexibility (1981).

Joint Flexibility

Examine the foot. A high arch indicates a tight heel cord and right joints. An average arch indicates average flexibility. Flat feet indicate loose joints and extreme flexibility (Marshall, 1981).

Shoulder Flexibility

While standing, ask clients to hold two ends of a tape measure with arms straight out at shoulder level; keeping the arms straight out, bring the tape above the head, then down behind the back, then forward again, using only as much tape as is necessary. Read the tape and use the following ratings: clients under 30 inches = looser than average; 30–40 inches = average; more than 40 = less flexible than average. For clients 25–45, add 5 inches to each measurement; for clients over 45, add 10 inches to each measurement (Marshall, 1981).

Thigh Flexibility

To assess thigh flexibility, ask clients to sit on the floor with back straight against the wall and bend their knees so the bottoms of their feet meet close to the groin. Measure the distance between the knees and the floor. For clients under 25 years of age, less than 4 inches is flexible; 4–7 inches is average; and more than 7 inches is tight. For clients 25–45 years, add 2 inches to each measurement; for clients over 45 years, add 2 inches more.

Heel Cord Flexibility

Ask the client to do the following: Lie down on the examining table or the floor. Extend the feet, keeping the knees straight. Flex the ankles and pull toes toward the shins.

Estimate the angle the foot makes to a line extending back through the heel. For all ages, over 105 degrees is flexible, 95–105 is average, and 95 degrees is tight.

Knee Flexibility

Ask clients to lean forward and touch the floor with knees straight and feet together. Delete this test for clients with back conditions. For clients under 25 years of age, less than 3 inches from touching the palms to the floor is flexible; 3–5 inches is average; 5 inches is tight. For clients aged 25–45, the measures are less than 4 inches, 4–7 inches, and more than 7 inches. For clients over 45 years old, the measures are less than 5 inches, 5–9 inches, and more than 9 inches (Marshall, 1981).

Table 19.2 provides information for assessing flexibility. Stretching exercises, weight lifting, yoga, and some touch therapies may assist clients to regain symmetry and flexibility.

FLEXIBILITY INTERVENTIONS

Based on the flexibility/tightness assessment, appropriate exercises can be chosen. Recommend endurance activities and patterned movements such as dancing, gymnastics, cycling, swimming, running, or walking for loose-jointed clients. They are more prone to ligament problems, partial dislocations, and knee problems. Recommend explosive activities such as basketball, hockey, tennis, racquetball, and sprinting for tight-jointed clients. They are most prone to muscle pulls and tears, torn ligaments and cartilage, lower back pain, tendonitis of the shoulder or elbow, and pinched nerves (Marshall, 1981). Figure 19.1 provides actions for enhancing flexibility in all clients.

Some movements devised by Moshe Feldenkrais (1977) can also improve flexibility (see: Chapter 25, Touch Therapies, for more information on Feldenkrais).

Enhancing Lower Back Flexibility

The following exercise can enhance movement and flexibility in the lower back:

> Lie on the floor with knees bent and feet flat on the floor. Cross the right leg over the left knee as if sitting in a chair with the legs crossed.

1–3 Reach left hand over shoulder and clasp right hand for 30 seconds and then switch arms.

4 Stand with feet 3 feet apart, and fingers laced behind back, palms up. Slowly lift arms up and over head while lowering the head gently towards the floor.

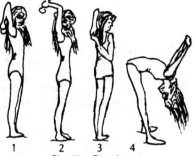

Shoulder Stretches

1–2 With legs wide apart, and palms on the floor, shift hips to the left, bending the left knee; then shift weight to the right, bending the right knee. Repeat 10 times each side in a slow, controlled motion.

3–4 Sit on the floor with soles of feet together; press with hands on the inside of the knees and hold for 30 seconds, then relax. Repeat 20 times.

Thigh Stretches

Place hands and feet on the floor, backside up; bend left knee and press right heel to the floor and hold, feeling the pull in the calf. Straighten left leg and bend right knee and press left heel to the floor and hold. Do 20 repetitions each side.

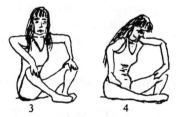

Heel Cord Stretches

Figure 19.1 Flexibility exercises. *(continued)*

1–2 Squat with palms on the floor directly under shoulders with head to knee; straighten legs, keeping palms and heels on the floor, then lower. Repeat 10 times.

3–4 Sit on the floor, one leg bent into opposite thigh, other leg straight out with foot flexed. Reach arms down the straight leg, lowering chest toward it. Bob very gently 15 times and then switch legs and repeat.

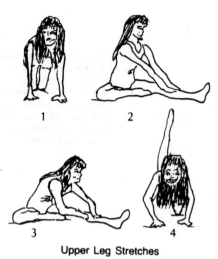

Upper Leg Stretches

Figure 19.1 *(continued)*

Extend arms out at shoulder level and let them relax. Continue breathing easily while slowly and smoothly letting the legs drop to the left toward the floor as far as possible and still be comfortable. Continue breathing. In a smooth continuous movement return legs to center and let them drop to the right toward the floor. With legs facing front, slowly place legs flat on the floor and observe the sensations in the lower back, pelvis, and legs. Lie still, breathing and noting changes and sensations.

Increasing Shoulder and Upper Back Movement and Flexibility

The following exercise is especially useful for individuals who sit for long periods of the day or for those who carry their tension in the upper part of their chest or back. Instruct clients to conduct the exercise as if in slow motion:

Table 19.2   Flexibility Assessments

Check off the items that best describe the client.

Flexibility area	Assessment
1. Body movement	_____ Moves as a solid block
	_____ Moves arms or legs freely, but not both
	_____ Walks with a spring in the step

Table 19.2 *(continued)*

Check off the items that best describe the client.

Flexibility area	Assessment
	_____ Walks gracefully
	_____ Arms swing in opposition to legs with knees bending, hips moving with legs, neck, and chest moveable
2. Thumb flexibility	_____ Angle between fingers and bent back thumb is more than 70 degrees (better than average)
	_____ Angle between fingers and bent back thumb is 60–70 degrees (average)
	_____ Angle between fingers and bent back thumb is less than 60 degrees (less than average)
3. Metacarpal-phalangeal extension	_____ more than 115 degrees (high)
	_____ 105–115 degrees (average)
	_____ less than 105 degrees (less than average)
4. Foot arch	_____ flat (extreme flexibility)
	_____ average (average flexibility)
5. Shoulder stretch	Under 25 years of age:
	_____ less than 30 inches (loose)
	_____ 30–40 inches (average)
	_____ more than 40 inches (less flexible than average)
	Age 25–40 years:
	_____ less than 35 inches (loose)
	_____ 35–45 inches (average)
	_____ 45+ inches (less flexible than average)
	Older than 45 years old:
	_____ 40 inches (loose)
	_____ 40–50 inches (average)
	_____ 50+ inches (less flexible than average)
6. Thigh stretch	Under 25 years of age:
	_____ less than 4 inches (loose)
	_____ 4–7 inches (average)
	_____ 7+ inches (tight)
	25–45 years of age:
	_____ less than 6 inches (loose)
	_____ 5–9 inches (average)
	_____ 9+ inches (tight)
	Age 45 and older:
	_____ less than 8 inches (loose)
	_____ 7–11 inches (average)
	_____ 11+ inches (tight)

(continued)

Table 19.2   *(continued)*

Check off the items that best describe the client.

Flexibility area	Assessment
7. Heel cord	_____ 105 degrees (flexible)
	_____ 95–105 degrees (average)
	_____ 95 degrees (tight)
8. Palms to floor with straight legs	Under 25 years of age:
	_____ less than 3 inches (flexible)
	_____ 3–5 inches (average)
	_____ 5+ inches (tight)
	25–45 years of age:
	_____ less than 4 inches (flexible)
	_____ 4–7 inches (average)
	_____ 7+ inches (tight)
	45 years of age:
	_____ less than 5 inches (flexible)
	_____ 5–9 inches (average)
	_____ 9+ inches (tight)

Lie on the floor, knees bent and feet flat on the floor. With arms extended and palms meeting each other in front, breathe comfortably and gradually allow the two arms to move toward the left at shoulder level. Move as far toward the floor as is comfortable. Continue breathing, letting the arms move in an arc over the body, directly over the nose and then toward the right side of the body at shoulder level. Continue breathing as the arms sweep to the left side and then return to the right side of the body. Use a very slow, continuous movement, paying attention to any points of resistance, relaxation, or tension. Note differences in the ability to carry out the movement on each repetition. When relaxation is attained, stop the movement and lie flat on the back, breathing easily and noting the effect on the body. When ready, slowly turn gradually onto the left side with the left leg on the bottom and the right leg bent at a 75–90 degree angle to the trunk. Find an angle of comfort. Continue breathing and slowly bend the right arm and move it across the body easing the arm effortlessly with the left palm on the right elbow, moving toward the right shoulder. Hold the position of an easy stretch and breathe easily. Continue holding the right arm and picture breathing into the shoulder as if there are tiny lungs located in the shoulder inhaling and exhaling as the client inhales and exhales. Continue to gradually stretch the right arm, using the left to support and assist in the stretch.

Holding the right hand in the left, gradually move the right arm to the right side of the body and back to the left side of the body, using one continuous movement. Continue breathing easily throughout. Lie flat on the floor on the back and note sensations in the upper and lower body as a result of the exercise. When ready, turn and lie on the left side of the body as before. Turn the right shoulder to the left side of the body, assisting with the right arm gradually and continuously, making sure to breathe comfortably. Hold the shoulder at the point of stretched comfort and move the left hand to the right shoulder. Hold the hand there and breathe into it, moving the left palm after several breaths to another spot on the shoulder when warmth is felt emanating from the shoulder. Close the eyes and imagine energy and warmth generating in the shoulder. Turn and lie flat on the back and note the effect. When ready, repeat all portions of the exercise using the right side of the body and the left shoulder. This series can also be completed while seated in a straight-backed chair. The opposite shoulder/arm is cradled in the other arm. A final component can be added while sitting. Place the left palm on the front of the right shoulder and gradually and firmly push the shoulder back as far as is comfortable while breathing deeply in and out. Hold in the extended position and picture tiny lungs breathing in and out at the point of pressure. Relax and note body sensations. Repeat with that arm several times and then repeat with the other shoulder.

Increasing Neck Flexibility

With age, the neck loses its flexibility, making it difficult to turn the head without turning the body, while driving or during other daily activities. Not only is this unsafe in some cases, but pain and discomfort frequently accompany the loss of neck flexibility. Suggest clients use the following movements to enhance neck flexibility:

While seated in a straight-backed chair, and keeping feet flat on the floor, let the right hand come up and over the top of the head. Let the fingers of the right hand rest comfortably a little below the left ear. Slowly and gradually, pull the head toward the right shoulder, silently asking the muscles of the neck and left chest to relax. Hold the head in a comfortable stretch. Repeat with the left arm.

AEROBIC EXERCISE

Aerobic exercise involves sustained, rhythmic activity of the large muscle groups. It uses large amounts of oxygen, causing an increase in heart rate, stroke volume, respiratory rate, and a relaxation of the small blood vessels leading to increased oxygenation.

The goal of aerobic exercise is to strengthen the cardiovascular system and increase stamina. Approximately 20 minutes of activity at the appropriate heart rate for each age range produces a training effect without straining the heart unduly. Aerobic exercise not only conditions the cardiovascular system, but it can also reduce body fat (Clark, 1996).

Benefits of Nonaerobic Exercise

Even exercise of moderate intensity for 30 minutes, or moderately vigorous physical activity accumulated over the course of a day, can lower the risk for the following conditions:

- heart disease
- high blood pressure
- type II, noninsulin-dependent diabetes
- obesity
- colon cancer
- arthritis
- bone loss

Regular moderate physical activity also can play a role in managing type I (insulin-dependent) diabetes and can contribute to weight and stress management (Prevention Report, 1994). Common moderate intensity activities, such as walking or cycling, climbing stairs instead of taking the elevator, or walking short distances instead of driving can contribute to the 30 minutes per day that is recommended (Pate et al., 1995).

Assessing Amount of Body Fat

Assess body fat by pinching the back of the upper middle arms. Use the following measures to assess amount of body fat.

- Less than 1/4 inches indicates a below average amount of body fat.
- 1/4–3/4 Inches indicates an average amount of body fat.
- More than 3/4 inches indicates a high percentage of body fat.

Other methods of determining body fat, in order of complexity and reliability, are calipers and water displacement. When using calipers, the skinfold sites commonly used are triceps, subscapula, suprailiac, and thigh (Clark, 1996).

CALCULATING A SAFE RANGE FOR AEROBIC EXERCISE

A safe range for aerobic exercise can be calculated by subtracting the client's age from maximum heart rate (220) + maximum attainable heart rate—resting heart rate x 0.6 and 0.8 + the resting heart rate.

e.g., $220 - 44 = 176 - 64 = 112 \times 0.6 = 67.2 + 64 = 131.2$
$112 \times 0.8 = 89.6 + 64 = 153.6$

In the above example, a 44 year-old person with a resting pulse of 64 needs to raise the pulse to between 131 and 154 to attain a conditioning effect. The pulse can be taken at intervals during exercise to ensure the safe range is not exceeded. Clients can be advised to take their pulse for 15 seconds and multiply by 4.

Pros and Cons of Stress Testing Prior to Starting an Exercise Program

Stress testing is most commonly accomplished by placing a client on a treadmill and using an electrocardiogram to measure the effects of strenuous running on heart activity. There are several reasons why stress testing may not be the best way to determine whether a strenuous exercise program can be safely undertaken.

1.   The stress test itself has a greater risk of precipitating a heart attack (risk level of 30%–60%) than does unaccustomed, severe exercise (risk level of 6%–12%). If clients gradually work up to a conditioning level, their risk should drop to less than one fifth the risk of a heart attack than if they have a stress test.
2.   The stress test is not a reliable indicator of persons at high risk for heart attack. False positives and false negatives abound. In a study of persons without symptoms of heart disease, 47% who tested "abnormal" on the stress test did not have heart disease; in another study, 62% of those who did have heart disease tested "normal" on the stress test (Vickery, 1978).

Reliable Indicators of Need for Medically Supervised Exercise

There are more reliable indicators that can be used to assess need for medical supervision prior to beginning an exercise program.

A "yes" answer to one or more of the following questions by someone over 35 years of age indicates a need for medical supervision:

1. Do you have any chest pain when you exert yourself?
2. Do you get short of breath with mild exertion?
3. Do you have pain in your legs when you walk, but not when you rest?
4. Do your ankles swell regularly (at times other than when menstruating)?

5. Has your health care practitioner ever told you that you have heart disease?

RECOMMENDING AN APPROPRIATE
AEROBIC EXERCISE REGIME

According to the National Exercise for Life Institute, there are several factors to consider when choosing an aerobic exercise:

1.   Is the exercise weight-bearing? Only weight-bearing exercise can prevent osteoporosis, but for clients who cannot tolerate weight-bearing due to pain or another condition, weight-bearing exercise may not be suitable.

2.   Is the exercise safe? Avoid any recommended exercise that puts undue strain or impact on the back, knees, or other joints. Immediate or delayed pain is a sign the exercise is not safe. Bicycling and running are examples of high-impact exercise.

3.   Is the exercise for the total body? An activity that uses both arms and legs provides the best cardiovascular benefit.

Walking, running, jogging, swimming, aquadynamics, and aerobic dance are examples of aerobic activities. Running and jogging are efficient, inexpensive approaches to increasing cardiovascular fitness. They can be started at any age, even by those who require rehabilitation. But, injuries of the ankle, knee, and lower back are common. Some can be prevented by using appropriate shoes (see Table 19.3), improving posture, and strengthening the abdominal and back muscles (see Table 19.4).

Table 19.3   Choosing a Running or Walking Shoe

Running shoe requirements	Walking shoe requirements
1/4"–1/2" lift or wedge; thick, soft heel; middle sole softer than outer sole to absorb shock of running on a hard surface; outer sole is flexible at the ball of the foot: test by compressing with the thumb; rounded toe to reduce blisters and allow room for toenails; feels comfortable first time on; heels should not slip; at least 1/4" extra room at front and sides of shoes	able to wiggle and spread out toes; sole flexes at the ball of the foot; should not have to be broken in; cushioned sole; arch support; leather and mesh upper; lightweight; curved sole to facilitate rolling heel-toe action of correct walking

Adapted from S. Hoag, *Choosing a running shoe* (1981); *The MN Wellness J* (July): 1–4; and G. Yanker, *The Complete Book of Exercise Walking* (1983). Chicago, IL: Contemporary Books.

Table 19.4 Improving Posture and Reducing Back Pain

Improving posture	1. Stand and move shoulders forward, then to the back, trying to touch the shoulder blades together (repeat 1–5 times). 2. Sit in am armless straight-backed chair. Hold arms at shoulder level with arms bent at elbows. Twist the body gently to the left and then the right several times (repeat 1–5 times). 3. Get on the floor on the knees. Shift weight back toward feet. Place hands out in front on the floor and walk the arms out, using fingertips, as if playing a vertical piano. If unable to get on the floor, stand facing a wall and walk the fingertips up and down the wall as far up as possible above head without incurring pain. 4. Stand with a chair in front, knees bent, and stomach muscles tight. Keep the shoulders and lower back still while tilting the pelvis back and forward (repeat 8–30 times, using a slow continuous movement). 5. Stand against a wall with knees slightly bent. Palms out, move arms from sides to meet at the top above the head (repeat 1–10 times, breathing freely throughout).
Strengthening lower back	1. While lying on back and keeping head on the floor, bring knees to chest and hold for a minute (repeat 1–5 times). 2. Kneel on all fours and alternately raise head and arch back like a lazy cat (repeat 1–5 times). 3. Lie on the floor and press pelvis to the floor and hold for 5 seconds (repeat 5–25 times). For soreness or stiffness, pretend the pelvis is a clock face and touch each hour clockwise and then counterclockwise. 4. While sitting on the floor, put one leg straight out and keep the other one bent to the side. Bend forward without straining and hold for 10 seconds to one minute, breathing into the stretch (repeat with other leg). 5. Sit in a chair and press the buttocks together, holding for 6 seconds. Relax and repeat. Build up to 20 times a day. 6. Stand with the back against a wall with feet a shoulder length apart. Slide down the wall to a crouch with knees bent to about 90 degrees. Count to 5 and slide back up the wall. Work up to 5 times. 7. Lie on the stomach with hands under shoulders, knees bent. Raise the upper part of the body, keeping hips and legs on the floor. Hold for 1–2 seconds, repeat up to 10 times, several times a day. 8. Lie on the back, knees bent and feet flat on the floor. Reach with head, shoulders, and hands toward or past the knees until abdominal muscles tighten, 5–100 times. 9. Stand behind a chair, hands on the chair back. Lift one leg back and up while keeping that knee straight. Return the leg slowly to the floor (repeat 5 times each leg). 10. Sit upright in a chair with legs straight out. Lift one leg waist high and return it to the floor (repeat 5 times each leg).

(continued)

Table 19.4 *(continued)*

11. Take the "ready" running position on the floor: crouch with right leg bent, weight on right foot and left leg out straight behind. Hold, then repeat with other leg.
12. Bend knees and crouch on floor. Put right leg out to the right in a 90-degree angle from left leg, then return to crouch (repeat with left leg).
13. Lie on stomach on floor or bed, head turned to one side and cradled on top of hands. Keeping legs and feet bent, move them gently to the right of the body and then to the left. (Uncross hands and re-cross with other hand on top; recradle head, turning it to the other side. Repeat leg movements.)

Adapted from: CC Clark, *Wellness Practitioner: Concepts, Research and Strategies*, New York, Springer Publishing Company, 1996.

Lower back pain affects 80% of the population at some time in their lives. Jogging, biking, paddling, rowing, baseball, and softball all put added strain on the back. Recommend another form of aerobic exercise if low back pain, previous injury, or poor jogging posture already exist.

Although jogging and running remain popular, walking is superior in several ways: fewer injuries are reported and walking is better for losing weight if brisk walking is maintained (1,012 calories per hour versus 782 calories per hour). The best way to differentiate brisk walking from jogging is that in walking, the feet are always on the ground, never in flight (Clark, 1996).

To improve walking technique, encourage clients to:

1. Hold the head and back erect, tighten the abdominal muscles, tuck buttocks under, and walk tall. Hold the image of a golden cord attached and pulling up from the upper chest.
2. Point the toes in the direction of travel, reaching out with hip, knee, and heel.
3. Plant the back edge of the heel of the forward moving foot at a 40-degree angle to the ground, setting the ankle slightly to the outside leg and foot at a 90-degree angle.
4. Pull forward with the leading leg while pushing back with the back leg.
5. Hold hands loosely clenched, arms at a 90-degree angle, just brushing the side. Move the arms as high as the chest in the front and near shoulder level in back. Inhale on the left arm swing, exhale on the right arm swing. Right arm moves forward with left leg and vice versa.
6. Focus eyes 10–15 feet ahead.
7. Check out nonparallel leg movements by walking in the snow, or sand, or observing. For a duck-footed walk, walk with a wider stance and practice walking on the heels. To correct pigeon-toed walking, exaggerate pointing the toes before the heel strikes and picture the toes pointing straight ahead. To correct favoring one leg, concentrate on the forward flow of the legs.

EXERCISE INTERVENTIONS WITH OLDER AND DEBILITATED ADULTS

Even nursing home residents can benefit from exercise. Fiatarone (1994) demonstrated that exercise training and multinutrient supplementation was beneficial for residents in a nursing home whose average age was 87.1 years. Probably the best exercise for clients of all ages and conditions is walking. If that is not feasible, most of the exercises can be adapted for use in a wheel chair or armchair. Even those who are severely debilitated can approximate some of the movements or at least rotate the wrists and ankles, flex and stretch wrists and feet, rotate the head toward the shoulders and exercise the face by exaggeratedly saying the vowels (A,E,I,O,U).

Feldenkrais' movements not only improve flexibility, but bring a new awareness to clients about their body movements and retrain movement in a more efficient manner. Masters and Houston (1978) suggested the following series to enhance leg and hip movement:

1. Sit halfway forward in a straight-back chair, legs spread a little wider than usual, knees bent, and feet parallel. Rest hands on the chair seat or side, not on the legs.
2. While breathing, let the right leg begin to drop slowly to the right, then bring it back to the middle, flat on the floor, paying attention to the sensation in the hip joint.
3. Extend the right leg out in front, resting the heel on the floor. Let the foot fall to the right, keeping the leg straight. Try it again, this time with the knee slightly bent. Repeat 20–25 times while breathing easily. Rest and observe the sensations in the lower body.
4. Extend the right leg in front, resting on the heel. Let the foot fall toward the left, keeping the leg straight. Let the foot gradually return to the middle. Try it again, this time with the knee slightly bent. Repeat 20–25 times while breathing comfortably. Rest and observe the sensations in the lower body.
5. While continuing to breathe throughout, and while holding the side of the chair for balance, extend the right leg and push the foot along the floor, keeping the leg straight, pushing off and back with the heel. Let the right side of the body follow the movement. Repeat the movement 20–25 times, noticing how the left shoulder goes back as the right shoulder moves forward.
6. Spread the feet and legs a little farther apart. Continue breathing comfortably while letting the right leg fall toward the left leg. Pay attention to the hip joint and right buttock as the leg falls. Put the right leg out a little farther in front and continue breathing and dropping the right leg toward the left leg. Watch as the leg moves and feel what happens in the hip joint and buttock.
7. Turn the right foot toward the left leg and then away from it. Notice the pressure on the left buttock when turning the right leg away from the left

leg. Let the whole body shift with the foot movement and pay attention to the body sensations. Repeat the movement 20–25 times while breathing. Rest.

8. Place the right foot parallel to the left foot and let the right leg flop from the left to the right. As the leg flops to the right, the foot will tilt on its right side. As the leg flops to the left, the foot will tilt on its left side. Experiment with different positions until the point where the leg moves most freely is found. Rest and breathe.

9. Shift the body weight onto the left buttock slightly so that the right buttock rises a little off the chair. Sink into the right buttock, and observe the left buttock rising off the chair. Repeat with the right buttock, noticing what happens in the hip joint during the movement. Remember to breathe on each movement.

10. Extend the right leg and foot off the floor an inch or two, while sitting way back in the chair. Make circles with the right foot, keeping the leg stiff and breathing easily. Make a few circles in the other direction, continuing to breathe throughout. Experiment with small circles, large circles, fast circles, slow circles. Rest.

11. Sit back in the chair with the right leg extended and the right foot a few inches off the floor. While breathing, move the foot and leg as a piece from left to right several times. Continue to breathe and flop the right foot left and right, keeping the leg straight. Rest and note body sensations.

12. Lean forward and extend the right leg, placing the heel on the floor. Slide the right foot backward and forward along the floor, keeping the knee straight. Note how differently the hip joint is now being used. Let the whole body move as the foot slides forward and back. Place the right hand on the right hip and feel the movement as the right foot and leg are moved to the right and to the left. Sense where the socket is that connects the leg into the hip and notice what is happening to the left side of the rib cage. Rest.

13. Place both feet side by side with the legs bent. Move the right knee from left to right and see how it moves. Breathe in as the right knee is moved from left to right. Breathe out and move the right knee from left to right. Note which way of breathing is easier. Repeat the movement, using the breathing (inhale or exhale) that is easier.

14. Extend both legs and lift the right leg several times and then the left leg several times. Note which leg feels lighter. Get up and walk around. Turn to the right and then to the left. Note in which direction it is easier to turn.

15. Lift the right leg and place it down in front of you. Then lift the left leg and place it in front of you. Note which leg made the larger movement. Rest and note the sensations in both sides and both legs.

16. Repeat numbers 1–15 using the left leg. Continue doing the exercise daily, alternating legs.

Table 19.5 provides exercise directions for bedridden clients.

Table 19.5 Exercises for Bedridden Clients

NOTE: Ask client to breathe throughout all exercises.

1. Raise the head from pillow as far as possible; add one raise of the head a week to a maximum of 10 repetitions.
2. Turn the head slowly to the left and then to the right; add one turn of the head per week to a maximum of 10 repetitions.
3. Shrug the shoulders up and back toward the ears as far as possible; add one repetition per week to a total of 10 repetitions.
4. Rotate the shoulders.
5. Bring the right arm (fully extended) over the head, left arm at side; bring down right arm to the side of the body and bring the left arm (fully extended) over the head. Work up to a maximum of 10 repetitions.
6. Cross the wrists at the abdomen and circle both arms at the same time, first clockwise and then counterclockwise; work up to 10 repetitions.
7. Clench the fists tightly and hold for several seconds, then extend the fingers and reach up as far as possible; work up to 10 repetitions.
8. Extend the arms forward and spread the fingers as far as possible; work up to 10 repetitions.
9. Make a fist and rotate the thumbs clockwise and then counterclockwise; work up to 10 repetitions.
10. Raise the right leg up as far as possible and return it to the bed; keep the leg as straight as possible without straining the lower back; work up to 10 repetitions each leg.
11. Grasp the right knee with both hands and very slowly pull it toward the chest while slowly moving the head toward the knee; work up to 5 repetitions with each knee.
12. Grasp both knees with both hands and very slowly pull them toward the chest while slowly moving the head toward the knees; work up to 10 repetitions.
13. With arms at sides of the body, slowly raise the head, shoulders, and legs several inches; hold, then return to lie flat; work up to 3 repetitions.
14. Extend both ankles toward the bottom of the bed; hold, then flex them toward the shins; hold, then relax. Work up to 10 repetitions.
15. Bicycle both legs slowly, completing up to 10 circles.
16. Lie on the stomach with chin resting on hands. Put heels apart and big toes together; squeeze the buttocks together as though trying to prevent a bowel movement; while squeezing, bring the heels slowly together and hold for 2–3 seconds, then relax on the bed. Work up to 5 repetitions.
17. Lie on the left side in a straight line and raise the left leg as high as possible over the other leg; hold, then return it to the bed. Work up to 10 repetitions. Turn on right side and raise left leg up to 10 repetitions.
18. Raise hips 5″–6″ off the bed, keeping arms at sides; hold several seconds, then relax into the bed. Work up to 5 repetitions.

Feldenkrais' movements can be used with older adults to enhance leg and hip movement (Masters and Houston, 1978):

1. Sit halfway forward in a straight-back chair, legs spread a little wider than usual, knees bent, and feet parallel. Rest hands on the chair seat or side, not on the legs.
2. While breathing, let the right leg begin to drop slowly to the right, then bring it back to the middle, paying attention to the sensation in the hip joint.
3. Extend the right leg out in front, resting the heel on the floor. Let the foot fall to the right, keeping the leg straight. Try it again, this time with the knee slightly bent. Repeat 20–25 times while breathing. Rest and observe the sensations in the lower body.
4. Extend the right leg in front, resting on the heel. Let the foot fall easily to the left, keeping the leg straight. Let it gradually return to the middle. Repeat as in no. 3 above.
5. While continuing to breathe throughout, extend the right leg and push the foot along the floor, keeping the leg straight, pushing off and back with the heel. Let the right side of the body follow the movement; hold the side of the chair for balance. As the movement is repeated (20–25 times), notice how the left shoulder goes back as the right shoulder moves forward.
6. Spread the feet and legs a little farther apart. Continue breathing regularly while letting the right leg fall toward the other leg. Pay attention to the hip joint and right buttock as the leg falls. Put the right leg out a little further in front and continue breathing and dropping the right leg toward the left leg and returning it to center. Watch as the leg moves and feel what happens in the hip joint and buttock.
7. Turn the right foot toward the left leg and then away from it; notice the pressure on the left buttock when turning the right leg away from the left leg. Let the whole body shift with the foot movement and pay attention to the body sensations. Repeat the movement while breathing for 20–25 times. Rest.
8. Place the right foot parallel to the left foot and let the right leg flop from the left to right. As the leg flops to the right, the foot will tilt on its right side; as the leg flops to the left, the foot will tilt on its left side. Experiment with different positions until the point where the leg moves the most freely is found. Rest and breathe.
9. Shift the body weight onto the left buttock slightly so the right buttock rises a little off the chair. Sink into the right buttock and observe the left buttock rising off the chair. Repeat right buttock, left buttock, noticing what happens in the hip joint during the movement and breathing on each movement.
10. Extend the right leg, foot off the floor an inch or so, sitting way back in the chair. Make circles with your foot, keeping the leg stiff, and breathing. Make a few in the other direction, continuing to breathe throughout. Experiment with small circles, large circles, fast and slow circles. Rest.

11. Sit back in the chair with right leg extended and foot off the floor a few inches. While breathing, move the foot and leg as a piece from left to right several times. Continue to breathe and flop the foot left and right, keeping the leg straight. Rest.

12. Lean forward and extend the right leg, placing the heel on the floor. Slide the foot backward and forward along the floor, keeping the knee straight. Note how differently the hip joint is being used now. Let the whole body move as the foot slides forward and back. Place the right hand on the right hip and feel the movement as the right foot and leg are moved to the right and to the left. Sense where the socket is that connects the leg into the hip and notice what is happening to the left side of the rib cage. Rest.

13. Place the two feet side by side with the legs bent. Move the right knee from left to right and see how it moves. Breathe in as the right knee is moved from left to right. Do the same movements while breathing out. Note which movement is easier. Repeat the movement using the breathing that is easiest. Rest.

14. Extend both legs and lift the right leg several times and then the left one. Note which feels lighter. Get up and walk around. Turn to the right and then to the left. Note in which direction it is easier to turn.

15. Lift the right leg in front and then the left leg; note which leg made the larger movement. Rest and note the sensations in both sides of your hip, and in both legs.

16. After a rest, or the next day, repeat nos. 1–15 above using the left leg. Continue doing the exercise daily, alternating legs.

OVERCOMING OBSTACLES TO EXERCISE

Although exercise is beneficial, clients can resist. Suggestions for helping clients make exercise a part of their lifestyle include:

1. Start small and keep it fun.

2. Keep records of daily and weekly progress; include both subjective reactions and objective measures such as weight, blood pressure, and pulse.

3. Focus on the rewards of exercise; keep a record of moods and compare differences in relaxation, energy, concentration, and sleep patterns.

4. Post goals, mottos, pictures of the ideal self, affirmations, and notes of encouragement.

5. Use visualization daily to picture successful attainment of exercise benefits, e.g., looking toned, radiant, graceful.

6. Work with a peer facilitator or join a structured exercise class, running club, or fitness center. Spend more time with people dedicated to wellness.

7. Reward and congratulate yourself for working toward exercise goals as well as attaining them. For example, after a month in an exercise program, buy a new pair of running shoes or treat yourself to a meal out.

8.   Use proper equipment and clothing when exercising.

9.   Include at least 10 minutes of warm-up and cool-down exercises in an exercise program. Avoid running up to the front door, going inside, and sitting down; complete stretching exercises, shower, and change to dry clothes.

10.   Stop exercising or at least slow down if any unusual, unexplainable symptoms occur.

11.   Avoid exercising for 2 hours after a large meal and eating for 1 hour after exercising.

12.   Vary exercise regimes to counter boredom.

13.   Walk or dance during lunch break and find other ways to work exercise into the daily calendar.

REFERENCES

Angotti C, & Levine MS. (1994). Review of 5 years of a combined dietary and physical fitness intervention for the control of serum cholesterol. *J Am Diet Assoc* 94:634–638.

Clark CC. (1996). *Wellness Practitioner, Concepts, Research and Strategies.* New York: Springer Publishing Company.

Feldenkrais M. (1977). *Awareness Through Movement.* New York: Harper and Row.

Fiatarone M. (1994). Exercise training and nutritional supplementation in very elderly people. *New Engl J Med* 330(25):1769–1775.

Kurtz R, & Prestera H. (1984). *The Body Reveals.* New York: Harper and Row.

Marshall J. (1981). How to get good looks, top performance and staying power for your body. *Self* March:56–72.

Masters R, & Houston J. (1978). *Listening to the Body.* New York: Delta.

National Headache Association. (1995). Exercise your headache away. *Let's Live* (February):81.

Pate RR, Rate M, Blair SN et al. (1995). Physical activity and public health: A recommendation from the Centers for Disease Control and the American College of Sports Medicine. *J Am Med Assoc* 273:402–407.

President's Council on Physical Fitness and Sports. n.d. *An Introduction to Running.* Washington, DC: National Institute of Health.

Prevention Report. (1994). Public Health Service. Office of Disease Prevention and Health Promotion. Washington, DC: U.S. Dept. Health and Human Services.

Shinton R, & Sagar G. (1993). Lifelong exercise and stroke. *Brit Med J* 307:231–234.

Vickery D. (1978). *Life Plan for Your Health.* Reading, MA: Addison-Wesley.

20

GUIDED IMAGERY

Imagery has been mentioned throughout most of recorded history. Hippocrates, the father of medicine, used it. Aristotle believed that images could change body functions, create illness, and assist healing. Freud believed that bringing images to consciousness was a basic growth process, and Jung was also convinced of the power of images (Epstein, 1989).

Everyone has had experiences with self-generated images: dreams, daydreams, and fantasies contain strong images generated by the right side of the brain. Imagery employs all six senses: visual, aural, tactile, olfactory, proprioceptive, and kinesthetic. Children have a well-developed sense of imaging. As they grow, this ability may lie dormant as the logical, rationale side of their brain is used in schoolwork and linear thought processes.

The power of imagery is derived from its right-brain source. This side of the brain, which controls the left side of the body, is primarily responsible for orientation in space, body image, artistic endeavor, and facial recognition. The right hemisphere is concerned with visual, holistic, intuitive, nonlinear thought, while the left side of the brain is involved with analytic, logical thinking, particularly verbal and mathematical functions (Ornstein, 1972).

Imagery allows direct access to the subconscious and autonomic nervous system functions. It bypasses the left brain and its tendency to try to solve problems through logical processing. Although useful in many situations, when logical processing goes awry, rumination and repetitive worrying occur, and stress increases. Imagery can bypass rumination to the essential core of issues, leading to effective problem solving, decreased anxiety, and increased healing potential.

The mind does not differentiate between an image of a situation and the actual experience. Practicing imagery in a relaxing safe environment provides experience that can be used in a stressful real-life situation. Positron emission tomography (PET) has demonstrated that the same parts of the cerebral cortex are activated whether imagining a situation or actually experiencing it (Rossman, 1993).

USES FOR GUIDED IMAGERY

There are four basic ways to use guided imagery with clients (Clark, 1996):

1. *Decreasing negative feelings.* When using guided imagery in this fashion, you can help clients identify feelings, dissatisfactions, tensions, and images that are affecting body functioning and change them to helpful elements.
2. *Healing.* When you use guided imagery for healing, you can help clients erase bacteria or viruses, build new cells to replace damaged ones, make rough areas smooth, hot areas cool, sore areas comfortable, tense areas relaxed, drain swollen areas, release pressure from tight areas, bring blood to areas that need nutrients or cleansing, make moist areas dry or dry areas moist, bring energy to fatigued areas, and enhance general wellness.
3. *Problem solving.* Used this way, clients learn to consult their intuitive sources of wisdom in a structured way or break down barriers to clear thinking.
4. *Preparing for upcoming situations.* By working back and forth between feeling relaxed and picturing a feared upcoming situation, clients can teach their bodies to stay relaxed in future situations.

Table 20.1 provides information on ways to use guided imagery with clients.

DECIDING WHEN TO USE GUIDED IMAGERY

When descriptions by clients are vivid enough that a picture can be formed, guided imagery may be the treatment of choice. It is a versatile approach that is often combined with relaxation therapy, music therapy, and hypnosis.

If clients are wary of the procedure or have difficulty obtaining a clear image, it may be useful to have them touch an object, then close their eyes and picture it. Another way to enhance imaging skill is to ask the client to view a movie, then close the eyes and picture a crucial scene.

CAUTIONS, COSTS, REIMBURSEMENT

Risks from using guided imagery are virtually nonexistent unless used in psychotherapy. In those cases, the practice should be restricted to trained psychologists, psychotherapists, or psychiatrists. There are minimal costs involved when using the procedure unless tape recordings are used. The only indirect costs are professional training time. When used with biofeedback or psychotherapy, significant costs can be incurred for professional services. Medical insurance plans are more likely to cover guided imagery if it is used for medical purposes (such as increasing circulation in Raynaud's disease), than for improving mood or enhancing coping ability (Post-White, 1998).

Table 20.1 Using Guided Imagery for Different Purposes

Purpose	Steps
Decreasing negative feelings	1. Help the client relax using either a taped relaxation exercise or see chapter 23, Relaxation, for in-session ideas.
	2. Ask the client to picture the painful or negative feelings.
	3. When the client has a vivid picture of them (size, shape, location, etc.) say, "Find a container . . . put all the anger (sadness, or whatever negative feeling) in the container, put a tight lid on it, and lock it tightly."
	4. When the feelings are locked up tightly, ask the client to "put the locked container in a place where it can no longer influence you." Clients may have difficulty with any of these steps and will often verbalize that they are not ready to give up their painful feelings yet.
Healing	1. Ask the client what area needs healing.
	2. Once a primary area has been identified, ask the client to "Go inside yourself" or "Imagine yourself very small and go inside and look at that area. What do you see?"
	3. Listen very carefully to what the client describes. If not much description is forthcoming ask, "What color is the area?" and "What temperature is the area?"
	4. Once color and temperature have been identified, ask the client to: "Make that area a healthy color," or "Make that dark area lighter," or "Make that red area a cool soothing color," or "Make that gray cold area pink and warm." A general rule is to prescribe the opposite of what the client describes.
Problem Solving	1. Help the client get to a relaxed position and state.
	2. Ask the client to "Tell me in three or four words what the problem is."
	3. Ask the client, "Are you ready to solve this problem?" If the answer is "yes" proceed to step 4; otherwise, select another problem.
	4. Picture the clearly defined problem in a bordered frame.
	5. See the solution in another frame, using a different color to create a border around the solution.
Preparing for upcoming situations	1. Ask the client to choose an upcoming, anxiety-provoking situation for practice.
	2. Assist client to attain a relaxed state.
	3. Ask the client to, "Imagine yourself as the director of a movie that you are going to run in your mind's eye. As director, you can stop or start the movie at any point that discomfort occurs. Picture everything about the situation: what is said, what you feel, what the other people say or do, smells, sounds, sensations—include it all. When you notice yourself becoming uncomfortable, stop the movie in your mind and go back to focusing on relaxing your body. When you're relaxed again, begin the movie a second before you became anxious. Work back and forth between relaxing and running your movie until you complete the whole scene and feel satisfied and relaxed."

USING GUIDED IMAGERY WITH CLIENTS

Using guided imagery effectively requires skill. Like other skills, if practitioners first practice the skill on themselves, they will gain a better understanding of its use (Post-White, 1998). Relaxing music can be used as a backdrop if the client agrees. It is thought to trigger emotional responses by directly influencing the limbic system (Lane, 1994).

The following guidelines are suggested for practicing guided imagery:

1. *Achieve a relaxed state.* Find a comfortable spot, uncrossing any extremities, and loosening tight clothes. Close your eyes and focus on breathing in your abdomen; say "in" on the inhale and "out" on the exhale. Experiment with breathing in a relaxing, healing color, allowing it to fill every part of your body. Clients who have difficulty relaxing can be read a relaxation script or listen to a relaxation tape. When relaxed, scan your body and fill any tense spots with relaxing, healing color.

2. *Imagine a safe, calming place.* In your mind, go to a place you enjoy—a place where you feel safe and comfortable. Picture that place vividly in your mind. Smell the smells of that place. Hear the sounds of that safe and comfortable place. Taste the tastes of your comfortable, safe place. Feel the feelings or sensations of that safe, comfortable place.

3. *Picture the part of you that needs healing.* Imagine that part looking healthy and working perfectly. (If it is tight or "tied in knots," imagine the knots loosening and the muscles spreading out, lengthening, widening. If the part is moist, see it drying up, and so on, always imagining the opposite of the problem area. An alternate is to imagine the area looking pink and healthy like its adjacent area or the other side or the other healthy appendage, whichever has meaning.)

4. *Reinforce imagery ability.* Remember that you can return to this place, these feelings, this way of being, anytime you want to, merely by picturing yourself as you are now. You can feel as you do now by letting your breathing move effortlessly to your abdominal area.

5. *Return to present.* When you are ready, come back through time and space, bringing with you all you've learned today, knowing the healing (problem solving, understanding) will stay with you always and can be enhanced merely by imagining yourself in this state of relaxed comfort in your favorite safe and enjoyable place. Open your eyes now, feeling relaxed and refreshed, ready to go about your daily activities (or ready to fall asleep and awake refreshed and relaxed).

WORKING WITH CHILDREN

Children as young as age three can use imagery. Since their boundaries between fantasy and reality are fluid, they can easily move into "Draw a picture of . . . " or "Let's pretend you are a . . . " or "Let's imagine . . . "

Older children may require a little more direction, e.g., "Let's use your imagination to . . . " or "Go into your imagination . . . " or "Let's use your imagination to change what's been happening."

Table 20.2 provides information for using guided imagery with specific conditions.

Table 20.2   Using Guided Imagery with Specific Conditions

Condition	Imagery
Abuse	Picture an abuse situation but this time bring an inner advisor, an angel, or a protector with you to protect you. Or, picture yourself going into a large house, find the Wounded Child and take her by the hand, telling her it's now safe to examine what happened to her. Enter the door labelled Pain and see what's inside. Enter the door labelled Fear and see what's inside. Enter the door labelled Guilt/Shame and finally, the door labelled Anger, experiencing the feelings in each of these rooms. Then, Adult and Wounded Child enter an empty room with a chair in the middle where Mom is seated, but remains silent while Child can say or do anything she wants. Mom leaves and Dad sits in the chair and Child says and does whatever she wants. Any other relevant adults are brought in and seated in the chair, one by one. Adult and Child go to the Room of Change and experience decision, free will, and change.
Aggressive, Acting out behavior	Picture your body as beautiful with a protective light around you and a little tube that connects you to happy memories that make you feel loving and kind. Picture another tube connecting to your heart that lets only loving things in and keeps you safe.
Anger	Picture the anger, allowing it to flow out of the body through your feet. When it has all flowed out, kick it away like a football, out over the edge of a cliff until it disappears.
Anorexia	Picture yourself in a mirror the way your subconscious sees you. Now, picture your image in a mirror the way you would like to see yourself. Now, slowly erase the picture your unconscious has painted and enlarge the image of the way you would like to see yourself.
Anxiety/ Borderline diagnosis	Picture a strong tree. Lean against it and feel its strength and support. Take this image with you and use it to feel relaxed and supported.
Blocks to changing	Picture that part of you that is concerned about moving on. Form an image of that part. When you have a clear image, ask that part of you what its concerns are. Negotiate with that part and find a way that part will agree to change.

(continued)

Table 20.2   *(continued)*

Condition	Imagery
Breech presentation (At least 2 weeks prior to delivery)	Picture the delivery, seeing your baby shift, turning around so that the head begins to move toward the birth canal first.
Cancer	Imagine your white blood cells are hungry fish, eating away at the weak, disorganized cancer cells. Or, picture a radiant light gently dissolving all your cancer cells. Or, picture the blood flow being turned off to all your cancer cells. Or, allow an image to emerge that represents your cancer. Give your image a voice and ask it what it wants and needs from you. Ask it what it might be protecting you from. Negotiate with the image to see if you can meet each other's needs. Or, contact your Inner Advisor. Ask that Advisor to give you healing advice. Or, picture an image that represents health and wellness and another of illness. Allow your wellness image to transform the illness image.
Confusion/ Unclear thinking	Picture yourself as a tree with roots growing out of your toes and fingertips, giving you a solid base of support.
Depression, Feeling trapped	Picture yourself in a cage. Picture yourself breaking out of that cage, doing whatever you have to do to get out.
Depression, Secondary to childhood abuse	Imagine that a Divine Being or Protector accompanies you, pointing out a solid floor for you to walk on and safe and secure passage.
Difficult people	Imagine a protective shield around you with an opening you control, letting in only positive energy.
Falling	Picture yourself walking confidently and feeling secure and safe.
Fatigue	Imagine an energy machine filling you with energy. You control the switch. Let the energy flow into your body.
Fear	Picture yourself behind a shield that protects you from all harm. Now, picture a situation you are afraid of, far far away from you, with you staying safe and protected behind your shield. When you are ready, bring the situation gradually closer, staying safe and calm behind your shield. Or, bring a Divine Being or Protector with you and picture the situation you fear. Or, picture all the fear in your body. Observe it, allowing the fear to rise, dissolve, change. Immerse yourself in it, breathing it in and out, seeing how easy it is to stay calm. For children: Use a "magic wand" to take away the fear or picture an inner advisor who knows exactly what to do to keep you feeling safe and calm.

Table 20.2 *(continued)*

Condition	Imagery
Headache	Picture your headache in your little finger rather than you head. Or, imagine yourself in a time and place where headaches do not exist.
Insomnia	Picture yourself when you had to stay awake, how tired you were, how much your eyes wanted to close, how you finally gave into your urge and fell into a deep, refreshing sleep.
Marital conflict	Picture a screen between you and your partner. Allow an image to form on that screen that depicts the problem you are having between you. Now, let that image fade and picture the solution to that problem forming on the screen.
Nightmares	Close your eyes and get back in the dream, taking your magic wand with you to change the dream so you are in total control of what happens.
Overweight	Picture your extra fat sitting on a chair next to you. Talk to your fat to see what is keeping it with you. What is the fat protecting you from? Find another image that brings you strength and power and impose that image over the fat image.
Pain	Picture the pain as a bird. Then ask it to fly away and nest far away. Or, picture the pain as a color, then turn the color into a liquid and let it drain out of the body, onto the floor, out the door and far, far away. Or, get in touch with the sensation of your body on the chair (couch, bed, floor). Picture a fist closed around your pain, slowly allowing your fingers to open and allow the pain to rest calmly in your palm. Observe it, allowing the pain sensations to arise, change, dissolve. Or, picture a time when time moved very slowly. Now, picture a time when you were having so much fun time flew by. Next time you have pain, imagine it passing by in a second.
Procrastination	Ask your unconscious mind to project images on your mental screen that show you how to save time and accomplish tasks.
Surgery	Picture yourself getting ready for surgery. You've had your medicine to relax and you are on your way to the operating room. As the anesthetic is given to you, you fall into a peaceful sleep. Picture yourself waking up after surgery with very little discomfort, healing quickly.
Suspicion/ Mistrust	Imagine a protective shield around you that allows only positive energy to affect you.

REFERENCES

Bresler D. (1992). Imagery and pain control. *Atlantis, the Imagery Newsletter* (October):1–2,4,8.

Carlson MJ. (1990). Working with the wounded child. *Atlantis, the Imagery Newsletter* (December):3,6.

Carlson MJ. (1991). Breaking out of the cage: Imagery and ritual. *Atlantis, the Imagery Newsletter* (June):3.

Gersten D. (1991a). Imagery with borderlines: In search of compassionate diagnosis. *Atlantis, the Imagery Newsletter* (February):1–2,4,8.

Gersten D. (1991b). Compendium of imageries for cancer. *Atlantis, the Imagery Newsletter* (April):5,7–8.

Gersten D. (1992). Embracing the pain. *Atlantis, the Imagery Newsletter* (October):5.

Gersten D. (1993a). Imagery and the family. *Atlantis, the Imagery Newsletter* (June):5–6.

Gersten D. (1993b). Dealing with difficult people. *Atlantis, the Imagery Newsletter* (April):3,7.

Gersten D. (1993c). Coping strategies for surgery. *Atlantis, the Imagery Newsletter* (August):3–4.

Gersten D. (1995). Working with resistance. *Atlantis, the Imagery Newsletter* (October):1–2,4,8.

Gersten D. (1995). The battlefield: Inner world of abuse, part II. *Atlantis, the Imagery Newsletter* (June):3,5–7.

Kutter L, & Stutzer C. (1996). Easing death's transition for children. *Atlantis, the Imagery Newsletter* (February):3–4,7.

Lane D. (1994). Effects of music therapy on immune function of hospitalized patients. *Quality of Life: A Nursing Challenge* 3(4):74–80.

Mehl L. (1993). Shamanic psychotherapy. *Atlantis, the Imagery Newsletter* (October):1–2,4.

Ornstein R. (1972). *The Psychology of Consciousness*. San Francisco: W.H. Freeman and Company.

Post-White J. (1998). Wind behind the sails: empowering our patients and ourselves. *Oncology Nursing Forum* 25(6):1011–1017.

Remen RN. (1992). Talking away the fat. *Atlantis, the Imagery Newsletter* (August):8.

Reznick C. (1994). Empowering kids through imagery. *Atlantis, the Imagery Newsletter* (April):5.

Rossman M. (1993). Imagery: Learning to use the mind's eye. In D. Goleman & J. Gurin (Eds.), *Mind/Body Medicine*. Yonkers, NY: Consumers Union.

21

HYPNOSIS

Hypnosis is a wakeful state of deep relaxation during which there is an alteration in the conscious level of thinking and remembering, and an increase in the ability to focus on a particular situation. Hypnosis is a heightened state of awareness that allows individuals to be more open to suggestion.

Most people have experienced a hypnotic state, e.g., when daydreaming or when concentrating intently on a book, movie, television program, or work project. A hypnotic state can occur while driving, too.

All hypnosis is really self-hypnosis because individuals will not accept a suggestion unless it fits with their value system. The self always remains in control. The practitioner works as a facilitator who provides the conditions under which an altered state can occur (Clark, 1996).

Hypnosis can be used to enhance wellness by resolving stammers, phobias, and facial ticks; changing habits such as smoking and overeating; reducing pain, depression, anxiety, sexual problems, alcoholism, speech disorders, memory/concentration, nausea, gastric hyperacidity, burns, skin disorders, Parkinsonism, headaches, asthma, and addictions (Clark, 1996; Klepser & Ostroff, 1998). Hypnosis will only work with clients who are ready to solve their problem (Rankin-Box, 1996).

Hypnosis can be helpful while clients are under anesthesia or in a coma. At that time, they are cognitively receptive and auditory input is directly absorbed. Clients undergoing surgery can listen (via headphones) to positive suggestions designed to minimize pain, promote healing, and hasten recovery (Klepser & Ostroff, 1998).

When using self-hypnosis as an intervention, the first step is to assist the client to a relaxed state. With practice, clients can learn to quickly relax and put themselves in a trance state.

RESEARCH BASE

Studies done decades ago demonstrate that hypnotic suggestion can alter some aspects of immunity. Other studies have shown that warts (virus-induced) can be removed by hearing and repeating a suggestion specific to removing warts while in a deeply relaxed, hypnotic state (Clark, 1996).

Sellick and Zaza (1998) reviewed the use of hypnosis for managing cancer pain. They found a great deal of support for its use in the management of pain related to cancer.

Defechereux and colleagues (1998) reported the use of hypnosis or anesthesia for surgery. They found that hypnosedation offered the same advantage as anesthesia. Twenty-one patients underwent a cervicotomy under hypnosedation for primary hyperparathyroidism. No conversion to general anesthesia was needed. Russo and colleagues (1998) used hypnosis to reverse a conversion disorder presenting as multiple sclerosis.

ASSESSING HYPNOTIZABILITY

Eighty to 90% of people can be hypnotized. Those who are severely emotionally disturbed, depressed, or suicidal respond more positively to psychotherapy than to hypnosis. Others who may not respond positively to hypnosis include: (1) individuals with psychosomatic conditions who deny any emotional component to their conditions, and (2) individuals who are neurologically impaired or mentally retarded, or who are in crisis (Clark, 1996).

Clients who are most likely to respond favorably to hypnosis include those who are: (1) highly motivated to learn hypnosis; (2) optimistic; (3) willing to try something new; (4) able to concentrate easily; (5) receptive to hypnosis; and, (6) imaginative. Even if clients do not have all of the above characteristics, they can learn hypnosis if they are willing to practice the technique frequently.

Clients are receptive to hypnotic suggestion when the following are present (Hadley & Staudacher, 1989):

1. relaxation;
2. sleepiness;
3. a rigidity or limpness in the muscles of the arms and legs;
4. skin warmth or coolness;
5. sensations of tingling or feelings of electricity;
6. narrowness of attention

THE INITIAL INTERVIEW

During the initial interview, use the steps that follow to identify your skills and brush up on needed education and practice so you will be helpful to clients (Hadley & Staudacher, 1989).

Needed Characteristics

To be an effective hypnotherapist, you must:

1. Treat each client as a unique individual.

2. Be able to identify problem areas, assess their severity, and determine the type of induction that would be useful.
3. Be able to identify and respond to clients' emotional needs.
4. Stay objective during a hypnotic session.
5. Keep your personal problems, aspirations, or values from influencing treatment.
6. Be accepting of and show ability to deal with emotional displays that may arise during hypnosis sessions.

Provide a Relaxing Environment

Use soothing music, soft colors, comfortable furnishings, and green plants to contribute to a sense of relaxing calm. Trouble-shoot potential sources of disturbance, especially noise, before a hypnotic session and circumvent them. If you cannot circumvent them, make any noises part of the relaxation. Wear neat, but casual clothes. Greet clients while you are in a relaxed and calm state; this will communicate to them that everything is under control and you are peaceful and competent. Use a relaxation exercise or self-hypnosis to prepare yourself for early sessions.

The First Interview

During the first interview, you need to do the following: listen for client motivation, define the problem, evaluate the effectiveness of hypnosis for each unique client, pinpoint problems and find alternatives, complete an induction, deal with special problems.

1. *Listen for motivation.* Clients may volunteer their motivation for using hypnosis. For those who don't, use the following statements to evoke motivation: "Why do you want to stop smoking? (lose weight, have more effective sleep, stop smoking, etc.)" "Is there any other reason that comes to mind?"
2. *Define the problem.* Find out the when, where, and why of the problematic behavior: "How often do you snack (binge, smoke, lose a night's sleep, etc.)?"
3. *Evaluate whether the client has unrealistic expectations regarding hypnosis.* Clients who may not be able to benefit from hypnosis include those who want to stop getting involved with the same kind of person, those who have bouts of deep depression, feel victimized and have simultaneous fears of engulfment and abandonment (borderline personality), and those who suffer from severe thought or mood disorders (psychotic or prepsychotic diagnoses).
4. *Help clients identify alternatives to the problematic behavior.* Elicit alternative behaviors to the problem from the client, e.g., "If you were under stress and chose not to eat a brownie, what would be the next best way to relax?"
5. *Complete an induction.* Either play a relaxation tape, read a relaxation script (see Relaxation Therapy, chapter 23), or follow the basic steps: notice

breathing; relax breathing; relax face and jaw; relax temples, eyes, eyelids; relax back of neck and shoulders; relax lower back; relax arms, relax chest; relax stomach; relax legs; relax feet and toes; count backwards from ten to one; imagine a special place; imagine peace, sense of well-being; positive feelings grow stronger; use appropriate suggestions (see below); coming back to this room, count one to three; feel great, alive, remembering all you've learned.

6. *Deal with special problems.* Anticipate questions or reactions and propose several solutions to each special problem.

THE USE OF SUGGESTION IN HYPNOSIS

For hypnosis to be effective, positive suggestions must be used. Suggestions are used all the time by the lay public and by professionals, but often they are in a negative form. Both negative and positive suggestions affect the subconscious mind, even when asleep or unconscious. Adverse suggestions, such as "She'll never come out of this alive," or "It's malignant, the patient doesn't have a chance," or "You can't be helped, you will have to learn to live with this condition," are heard and acted upon by the hearer. Although the last comment seems innocuous, taken literally, it means the client will die if the symptom is lost (Clark, 1996).

Suggestions are most effective and wellness-enhancing when phrased in a positive form, e.g., "I will feel comfortable and confident during the interview tomorrow," (as opposed to "I will not feel tense tomorrow."). Formulating suggestions in the becoming mode is often very effective, e.g., "My comfort is gradually increasing." The best results occur when only one or two suggestions are used. Bombarding a client with numerous suggestions can dilute all of them.

Suggestions can be used to reduce stress related to smoking, drinking, overeating, taking harmful drugs, destructive anger, timidity, anxiety, allergies, itching, asthma, anger, study problems, and pain. The basic self-hypnosis state is induced, but the suggestions differ based on the stressor. Suggestions are usually said aloud, but they can also be placed on an audiotape or written and then read aloud.

Suggestions can be direct ("Your body is feeling more and more relaxed") or indirect ("You may notice that your body can feel more and more relaxed.") Indirect suggestions have a greater chance of being effective because just noting a change is defined as an appropriate response. Indirect suggestions are called "fail-safe" because any response that is evoked is considered positive (Larkin, 1990).

Likewise, making any external noises part of the relaxation response can lead to deeper relaxation. It is preferable to hold hypnotic sessions in a quiet, private place, but when that is not possible, simply suggest to the client: "Make any external noises part of the relaxation process."

Types of Suggestions

Permissive comments also facilitate relaxation, e.g., "You might be surprised to discover . . . " or "Perhaps you've already noticed . . . " *Contingent suggestions* link something that is uncontestably true with a hoped for response, e.g., "As you inhale (an undeniable fact), you can begin to notice how much more relaxed you feel." *Conjunctive suggestions* also link indisputable fact with hoped for responses, but use the word "and" to link them, e.g., "You're sitting in the chair and you can notice something pleasantly different happening to your right foot." *Conversational postulates* use questions to direct behavior, e.g., "Can you find a comfortable spot on the wall to focus on?" *Dissociative postulates* separate perception of body parts, e.g., "While that arm over there continues to heal, you can rest comfortably in the chair," or "Take your mind to a pleasant and relaxing spot while I take care of that burn on your hand." *Interspersed suggestions* use direct suggestion within the framework of conversation, e.g., "You can keep on relaxing Emma, while I take a look at this wound," or "I enjoy lying on the beach, too, Tom, it feels so comfortable, just lying there, feeling the warm sun on my face and arms." *Posthypnotic suggestion* used during hypnosis is intended to be carried out in the subsequent waking state, e.g., "When the nurse practitioner comes to remove the stitches, you can be surprised at how quickly you relax and feel comfortable" (Larkin, 1990).

Use of the Hypnotic Voice

The voice alone can elicit a trance state. The two most useful kinds of verbal presentation for inducing a trance are a monotone voice and a rhythmic or singsong voice. Use a monotone voice without inflection or variety in pitch or volume. A rhythmic voice stresses words in the sentence, e.g., *deep*er, *deep*er, into total relaxation. Practice one or both voices and find which one works best for you.

Other elements in basic delivery can also enhance a trance. The following elements can be used alone or combined for more powerful trances: (1) Word distortion for emphasis and reinforcement, (2) Raised pitch, (3) Uninterrupted rhythm, and, (4) Pauses.

Emphasize words to achieve a special effect, e.g., feel your muscles *widen and lengthen* as they *relax, loosen,* and let go. Raised pitch penetrates a relaxed state and is used to end an induction, e.g., "one, two, three, *open your eyes, feeling relaxed and refreshed.* Pitch can also provide posthypnotic suggestions, e.g., "Feeling relaxed and open to change and *now you will stop smoking forever.*" Connective words such as "and" are used to provide an uninterrupted rhythm, e.g., "You feel yourself relaxing more and more and just relaxing so much that the next time you inhale you feel a hundred times more relaxed . . . "

Pauses allow the client time to respond to a suggestion, e.g., "Take a deep breath (pause for 3 seconds) and inhale relaxation and comfort, perhaps as a soothing color (pause for 3 seconds) . . . " Pauses also allow time for clients to get into a relaxed state, e.g., "Let the relaxation flow, filling your scalp and hair with relaxation (pause for 3 seconds) . . . inhale again and let the relaxation flow across your forehead (pause for 3 seconds), eyebrows (pause for 3 seconds) . . . "

It is absolutely necessary to allow adequate time for each response. Your feelings of relaxation can guide you. If you are beginning to relax and feel almost at a trance state yourself, you are probably using the right amount of pauses and other hypnotic voice techniques. If you do not feel relaxed and find yourself hurrying and feeling anxious, practice more pauses, more of a monotone, more connective words, etc.

Use Table 21.1 to choose individualized objectives for clients.

GUIDELINES FOR EFFECTIVE SUGGESTIONS

Formulate suggestions using the following guidelines (Hadley & Staudacher, 1989):

1. Make direct, simple, and concise suggestions ("When I count to three, you will go back in time to your first experience in an elevator.").

2. Repeat suggestions, e.g., "You have stopped smoking, stopped smoking, you no longer smoke."

3. Keep suggestions believable and desirable by consulting with clients about their goals, e.g., "What do you believe you are capable of doing that you want to do?"

4. Create a time frame for suggestions, e.g., "In a moment, you will raise the index finger of your right hand to indicate you are totally relaxed," or "Every morning you will arrive on time for work."

5. Choose suggestions that can be interpreted literally, e.g., "Today when you leave work, you will turn off the lights in your office, and drive home feeling relaxed and comfortable." Ordering the suggestion in a different order could create problems for your client.

Table 21.1   Suggestion Objectives for Working With Clients

Objective	Suggestion
To elicit a physical response	"Feel your legs growing heavier and heavier . . . "
To deepen a hypnotic trance	"Let your mind and body drift deeper into relaxation with every breath you take" or "Feel the sensations of your back against the chair, the bottoms of your feet on the floor . . . "
To create imagery	"Picture yourself in a wide, green peaceful meadow."
To alter behavior	"You are now a nonsmoker, you have no wish to smoke."

6. Limit suggestions to one problem area at a time, e.g., do not combine a suggestion on smoking cessation with one on weight loss.

7. Break down major goals into a series of incremental steps, e.g., "All week, you will avoid yelling at people who cut you off while you're driving." In the next weeks, progress step-by-step until the client can smile when someone cuts her off.

8. Use positive words in formulating suggestions, e.g., "You can . . . ", "You are already . . . ", "You will . . . ", "You are . . . "

9. Keep suggestions as general as possible to avoid negative memories, e.g., "Relax and float in a deep state of relaxation," not "Relax and imagine yourself as a child floating in a rubber raft on a lake."

10. Use cue words or phrases to trigger and emphasize suggestions, e.g., "After you have eaten one small plate of food, you will feel *full* and no longer in need of food," or "As you drive home after work, say your cue word, 'open' to keep comfortable and relaxed," or as you walk into a room of strangers, say the word 'Queen Elizabeth' to yourself and feel confident and full of self-worth."

11. Ask the client to select an image that is meaningful to his or her goal, e.g., "Picture yourself at work looking and feeling calm and relaxed," or "Picture yourself at your perfect weight."

12. Use imagery that evokes all the senses: sight, sound, touch, smell, and taste, e.g., "See all the sights associated with _____, hear all the sounds associated with _____, feel all the sensations associated with _____, smell all the smells associated with _____, and taste the tastes associated with _____.

13. Safeguard against any unwanted suggestions that may be left after an induction by suggesting, "You will return to your usual state and reject all suggestions that are not related to areas of self-improvement and healthy functioning."

BASIC INSTRUCTIONS FOR SELF-HYPNOSIS

Table 21.2 provides basic instructions for self-hypnosis.

CAUTIONS

The practitioner must practice with simulated clients prior to working with real-life clients, identifying problematic areas of the process from induction to ending. Avoid using hypnosis for long-standing problems that may require additional counseling expertise. If clients report feeling light-headed, ask them to "Ground yourself by picturing yourself as a tree with roots growing out of your toes and fingertips into the earth, giving you a solid, substantial base." It clients fall asleep

Table 21.2   Basic Instructions for Self-Hypnosis

Phase of Hypnosis	Interventions
Induction	Use a relaxation technique to induce a trance that fits with the client's belief system Use linkages to fact, e.g., "As you breathe in and out (fact), you'll feel more and more relaxed."
Trigger	Use a word, symbol, or image that can deepen relaxation, e.g., "The next time you inhale you will be a thousand times more relaxed," or, "The next time you see a cigarette, you will have no interest in smoking it."
Deepening	Use a count that goes from 10 to 1, e.g., "Imagine a beautiful staircase with 10 steps and the 10 steps lead you to a special and beautiful place. I'm going to count from 1 to 10 and imagine taking 10 steps up, and as you take each step, relax even more deeply, one, relax even deeper, two . . . "
Ideo-motor response	Prior to beginning, agree on an ideo-motor response the client can use to indicate level of relaxation, e.g., "Raise the index finger of your right hand when you feel completely relaxed; raise the index finger of your left hand if you begin to lose your sense of relaxation."
Therapy	Address the client's concerns, e.g., "You are beginning to feel (see yourself) more relaxed in business meetings." Use positive statements and set positive expectations that can be met, e.g., "After surgery, expect to sit, walk, and eat comfortably within 6 hours or less."
Lightening/ Reorientation	"You're coming back to this room, keeping your eyes closed, but knowing that any time you want to be in hypnosis, you only need to close your eyes and picture yourself in this chair, in this room, totally relaxed."
Ending	"I'm going to count to three. When you hear the word 'three' you will open your eyes, bringing back with you everything you learned today, keeping with you that sense of relaxation and peacefulness. One. Two. Three."

during a trance, gently, but firmly, ask them to, "Wake up now, opening your eyes when I count to three, feeling relaxed, refreshed, and wide awake."

USING HYPNOSIS WITH CLIENTS

The following steps need to be taken when using hypnosis with clients.

1.   Obtain training in the use of hypnosis with clients. Continuing education and certification programs are available. (See Appendix.)

2.   Take a general history from the client, identifying the problem(s) of current concern and identifying positive suggestions, based on the client's words, to be used during treatment.

3.   Agree on ideo-motor responses the client will use to indicate relaxation while under hypnosis.

4.   Use a relaxation technique to evoke a trance. (See chapter 23 for suggestions.) Choose a trance induction that suits the client. Use a walk along the beach or a trip to the mountains assuming these situations are relaxing. The best approach is to ask clients what is relaxing for them, or ask them to imagine a scene in which they would feel relaxed (Rankin-Box, 1996).

5.   Use a monotone voice and repeat important suggestions and phrases numerous times, interspersing the words, "relaxed," "comfortable," "confident," "calm," etc., throughout the session.

6.   Bring clients back from hypnosis gradually, reorienting them to being in the present time and space.

7.   Tell clients that they will open their eyes when you count to three and that they will feel relaxed, refreshed, and confident.

REFERENCES

Clark CC. (1996). *Wellness Practitioner, Concepts, Research and Strategies.* New York: Springer Publishing Company.

Defechereux T, Faymonville ME, Joris J, Hamoir E, Moscato A, & Meurisse M. (1998). Surgery under hypnosedation. A new therapeutic approach to hyperparathyroidism. *Ann Chir* 52(5):439–443.

Hadley J, & Staudacher C. (1989). *Hypnosis for Change.* Oakland, CA: New Harbinger Publications.

Klepser C, & Ostroff B. (1998). Hypnotherapy. *The Nursing Spectrum* (September 21):4–5.

Larkin DM. (1990). Therapeutic suggestion. In R. Zahourek (Ed.), *Therapeutic Suggestion in Patient Care.* New York: Brunner/Mazel.

Rankin-Box D. (1996). Hypnosis. In VE Slater, and DF Rankin-Box (Eds.), *The Nurses' Handbook of Complementary Therapies.* New York: Churchill Livingstone.

Russo MB, Books FR, Fontenot J, Dopler, BM, Neely, ET, and Halliday, AW. (1998). Conversion disorder masquerading as multiple sclerosis. *Military Medicine* 163(10):709–710.

Sellick SM, & Zaza C. (1998). Critical review of 5 nonpharmacologic strategies for managing cancer pain. *Cancer Prev Control* 2(1):7–14.

22

MEDITATION

Meditation is a self-directed practice that is used to relax the body and calm the mind. During the practice of meditation, the mind settles down into a silent state, and the body's internal mechanisms repair the body, providing physiological benefits including: synchronous alpha, theta, and beta waves as indicated by electroencephalogram (EEG); light and/or suspended breathing pattern; decreased heart rate; decreased plasma cortisol, TSH, and lactate; increased plasma prolactin and phenylalanine; redistribution of blood flow away from the abdomen and toward the brain (Wallace, 1986). Meditation has been utilized to reduce stress and anxiety, to enhance general well-being, and to expand awareness (Miller, Fletcher, & Kabat-Zinn, 1995; Kreitzer, 1998).

TYPES OF MEDITATION

Transcendental Meditation

The most well-known type of meditation is called *transcendental meditation* (TM). It is the process of focusing on a thought or word, called a *mantra*, until attention transcends its common meaning. As a result of this focus, subtler meanings of thought are perceived. It is believed that *prana*, the cosmic vibratory energy of the universe, connects the individual to a transcendental existence during which slow, rhythmic nasal and abdominal breathing prevail (Fried & Grimaldi, 1993). Unlike breathing exercises, in TM breathing is not guided. There is no attempt to interfere with breathing. It is simply allowed to happen.

Centering Prayer

Centering Prayer is another kind of meditation, but is more Christian-based. This type of meditation is designed to withdraw attention from the ordinary flow of thoughts by focusing on a sacred word (Keating, 1995).

Relaxation Response

The relaxation response includes four elements that produce its effects. A *quiet environment* is used to help individuals concentrate on a mental device by eliminating outside distractions, including music. Clients are encouraged to use the same quiet environment each time meditation is practiced so that there is no need to adjust to new surroundings.

Finding a *comfortable position* and maintaining it during meditation contributes to the relaxation response. Sitting in a chair may be preferred, since sleep often results if the meditator lies down.

A *mental device* is used to shift the mind from logical thought to inner rumination. The mental device can be a sound, word, phrase, or focal object. If words are used, they are repeated either silently or aloud whenever meditation is practiced. If an object is used, it is focused on during the meditative practice.

A *passive attitude* is the most important element in eliciting the relaxation response. This is more difficult than it seems. Distracting thoughts and images often occur during meditation and clients need to be counseled to let thoughts and images happen (Benson, 1975).

Mindfulness Meditation

Mindfulness meditation describes the Buddhist practice of *vipassana* meditation. The goal is to be a detached observer of internal mental processes. The stream of thoughts, feelings, drives, and images that occur are focused on in turn without being considered an intrusion.

Meditation in action is an extension of mindfulness (Borysenko, 1988). The here-and-now becomes the focus for meditation in this approach. The client stays in a relaxed state while attending to activities in his or her inner and outer worlds.

RESEARCH BASE

A number of psychophysiological changes occur during TM, including slower breathing; lower ventilation volume, heart rate, and blood pressure; and a change in the EEG power spectrum, with an increase in the alpha band and transient theta (Badawi et al., 1984; Shapiro, 1982; *Scientific Research on Transcendental Meditation,* http://www.tm.org, accessed 1998).

Although meditation alone may not be sufficient to lower severe or moderately high blood pressure, it can reduce the amount of antihypertensive medication needed. Additionally, the practice of meditation may help prevent hypertension (Benson, Rosner, Marzetta, & Klemchuk, 1974; Pollock, Weber, Case, & Laragh, 1977).

Kabat-Zinn, Lipworth, and Burney (1985) reported on the use of meditation for chronic pain. They used a type of meditation called mindfulness. Statistically significant reductions in the following indicants were noted: present-moment pain; negative body image; inhibition of activity by pain; anxiety and depression; and, drug utilization. Overall increases in feelings of self-esteem and activity levels were also found. Improvements for all measures were maintained at a 15-month follow-up after meditation training, except for present-moment pain. Additionally, the majority of participants reported they had made meditation practice part of their daily regime.

Kabat-Zinn and colleagues (1998) also reported the use of mindfulness meditation for stress reduction in individuals with psoriasis and for anxiety (Miller, Fletcher, & Kabat-Zinn, 1995). Singh and colleagues (1998) reported the use of meditation, education, and movement therapy. An 8-week combined intervention with 20 individuals diagnosed with fibromyalgia resulted in a significant reduction in pain, fatigue, and sleeplessness, and improved function, mood state, and general health.

The following major areas of research have shown significantly positive results: figural and verbal creativity, improved moral behavior and advanced ego development, decreased anxiety, improved self-esteem, decreased admission to psychiatric hospitals, decreased substance abuse (cigarettes and addictive drugs), decreased criminal behavior, decreased blood pressure, decreased blood cholesterol, increased DHEAS, increased life expectancy, and decreased medical care utilization (*Scientific Research on Transcendental Meditation*, http://www.tm.org).

GUIDELINES FOR TEACHING CLIENTS MEDITATION

Use the following guidelines to teach clients to meditate (Benson, 1975; Everly & Rosenfeld, 1981; Lazarus, 1976):

1. Choose a time to meditate that is at least 2 hours after eating. (Digestion interferes with meditation.)
2. Select a quiet place where you will not be disturbed.
3. Sit in a comfortable position in a chair with a straight back.
4. Close your eyes.
5. Use a relaxation exercise to prepare for meditation. (See chapter 23.)
6. Focus on your breathing, allowing the breath to go in and out effortlessly.
7. Repeat your focus word (or symbol) or focus on your chosen object for at least 20–30 minutes for each meditation session.
8. Meditate at least daily, preferably twice a day.
9. Understand that it may take 6–7 teaching sessions to learn meditation and that about a month of practice will be needed before significant mind/body changes occur (Benson, 1975; LeShan, 1974; Credidio, 1982; Lehrer, Shoicket, Carrington, & Woolfolk, 1980).
10. Avoid meditating if any of the following occur: light-headedness, hallucinations, depression, suicidal thoughts.

11. If taking any medication, discuss the effects of meditation on dosage. (Meditation frequently results in needing a smaller dosage of insulin, sedatives, and cardiovascular medications.)

REFERENCES

Badawi K, Wallace RK, Orme-Johnson D, & Rouyere AM. (1984). Electrophysiologic characteristics of respiratory suspension periods during the practice of the transcendental meditation program. *Psychosom. Med.* 46:267–276.

Benson H, Rosner B, Marzetta B, & Klemchuk H. (1974). Decreased blood pressure in pharmacologically treated hypertensive patients who regularly ellicited the relaxation response. *Lancet* 1:289–291.

Benson H. (1975). *The Relaxation Response.* New York: Avon.

Borysenko J. (1988). *Minding the Body, Mending the Mind.* New York: Bantam.

Credidio S. (1982). Comparative effectiveness of patterned biofeedback vs. meditation training on EMG and skin temperature changes. *Behavior Research and Therapy* 20:233–241.

Everly G, & Rosenfeld R. (1981). *The Nature and Treatment of the Stress Response.* New York: Plenum.

Fried R, & Grimadli J. (1993). *The Psychology and Physiology of Breathing.* New York: Plenum.

Kabat-Zinn J, Lipworth L, & Burney R. (1985). The clinical use of mindfulness meditation for the self-regulation of chronic pain. *Journal of Behavioral Medicine* 8(2):163–190.

Kabat-Zinn J, Wheeler E, Light T, Skillings A, Scharf MJ, Cropley TG, Hosmer D, & Bernhard JD. (1998). Influence of a mindfulness meditation-based stress reduction intervention on rates of skin clearing in patients with moderate to severe psoriasis undergoing phototherapy (UVB) and photochemotherapy. *Psychosom Med* 60(5):625–632.

Keating T. (1995). *Open Mind, Open Heart.* New York: Continuum Publishing.

Kreitzer MJ. (1998). Meditation. In M Snyder and R Lindquist (Eds.), *Complementary/ Alternative Therapies in Nursing.* 3rd ed. New York: Springer Publishing Company.

Lazarus A. (1976). Psychiatric problems precipitated by transcendental meditation. *Psychological Report* 39:601–602.

Lehrer P, Schoicket S, Carrington P, & Woolfolk R. (1980). Psychophysiological and cognitive responses to stressful stimuli in subjects practicing progressive relaxation and clinically standardized meditation. *Behavior Research and Therapy* 18:293–303.

LeShan L. (1974). *How to Meditate.* Boston: Little, Brown.

Miller J, Fletcher K, & Kabat-Zinn J. (1995). Three-year follow-up and clinical implications of a mindfulness meditation-based stress reduction intervention in the treatment of anxiety disorders. *General Hospital Psychiatry* 17:192–200.

Pollock A, Weber M, Case D, & Laragh J. (1977). Limitations of transcendental meditation program. *Psychosom Med* 49:493–507.

Scientific Research on Transcendental Meditation. http://www.tm.org.

Shapiro BA, Harrison RA, & Walton JR. (1982). *Clinical Application of Blood Gases.* 3rd ed. Chicago: Year Book Medical Publishers.

Singh BB, Bermna BM, Hadhazy VA, & Creamer P. (1998). A pilot study of cognitive behavioral therapy in fibromyalgia. *Altern Ther Health Med* 4(2):67–70.

Wallace RK. (1986). *Neurophysiology of Enlightenment.* Fairfield, IA: MIU Press.

23

RELAXATION THERAPY

The body responds to anxiety-provoking thoughts and events with muscle tension. Physiological tension increases the subjective experience of anxiety. Relaxation of the muscles through Relaxation Therapy reduces pulse rate and blood pressure and decreases perspiration and respiration rates.

There are a number of techniques that can assist in relaxation and enhance change toward wellness. Relaxation techniques have been found useful in the treatment of muscular tension, anxiety, insomnia, depression, fatigue, irritable bowel, muscle spasms, neck and back pain, high blood pressure, phobias, and stuttering (Davis, McKay, & Eshelman, 1995).

Most individuals are not aware when their muscles are chronically tense, let alone anticipate how the constriction may be affecting their circulation, movement, or tendency to develop chronic illness or discomfort. When the practitioner is in a relaxed state, working with a relaxed client, both are more open to one another, and can listen and learn more easily (Clark, 1996).

RESEARCH BASE

Sharma and colleagues (1998) evaluated the influence of a 5-week relaxation therapy on the state of individuals with borderline hypertension. The study group consisted of 30 clients with high blood pressure. The study-makers observed significant change in anxiety, defensiveness, self-confidence, introspection, nurturance, affiliation, heterosexuality, change and succorance scales.

Timmerman and colleagues (1998) combined relaxation therapy with several other treatments on individuals in the community without serious mental health complaints, but with an increased chance of developing them as a result of stress. Potential participants were randomly selected from the community at large and then screened for the training program. The control group consisted of individuals with a similar risk profile as those in the training group, but they did not take part in the training. The training group received instruction in several stress-management techniques: changing unhealthy lifestyle, relaxation training, problem-solving training, and social skills training. Multivariate analyses of variance showed that the training group, as compared to the control group, reported significantly less distress, less trait anxiety, fewer daily hassles, more assertiveness, and more satisfaction with social support at follow-up. There were, however, no significant changes found in the coping skills of the training or the control group.

Penava and colleagues (1998) reported on the use of relaxation training with cognitive restructuring and diaphragmatic breathing. They examined the rate of symptom improvement in individuals with panic disorder in an outpatient clinic setting. Treatment included a standard program of 12 sessions that emphasized information, interoceptive and situational exposure, and cognitive restructuring. Individuals achieved significant gains on all panic disorder dimensions assessed, with the largest reduction of symptoms during the first third of treatment.

Coldwell and colleagues (1998) reported on the use of a computer program for reducing dental fear—CARL, the Computer Assisted Relaxation Learning program that presented a video-taped exposure hierarchy and scripts for a practitioner to use with clients. A one-year follow-up of participants in a placebo-controlled clinical trial showed all participants were able to receive two dental injections and reduce their general fear of dental injections.

TEACHING RELAXATION SKILLS

Relaxation is a skill. Like other skills, it requires practice to achieve mastery. Table 23.1 presents several types of relaxation exercises that can be used with clients (Clark, 1996).

CASE STUDY

Mr. Gordon, age 50, was president of his own computer programming company. He was working on a Ph.D. in health services and was supporting two young adult children in college. He came to the practitioner's office complaining of back pain, digestive upset, inability to sleep, and TMJ. He told the practitioner his family nurse practitioner had "run all the tests and she says there is no organic cause of my symptoms. Can you help me?"

The complementary practitioner started a Relaxation Therapy program, including having Mr. Gordon help develop his own relaxation tape to use between sessions. At the end of 3 weeks on the program, Mr. Gordon reported a decrease in symptoms. After 10 weeks, Mr. Gordon and the practitioner terminated their sessions. On follow-up 6 months later, Mr. Gordon was still using the relaxation tape and only had minor symptoms during acute stress situations.

Table 23.1   Relaxation Exercises

Progressive Relaxation

1. Lie down in a comfortable spot or sit in a comfortable chair.
2. Close your eyes. Follow steps 3–10, tensing for 5–7 seconds and relaxing for 20–30 seconds. Allow yourself to deeply experience bodily changes.
3. Tense all the muscles of your hands, forearms, and upper arms.
4. Let all the tension out of the muscles of your hands, forearms, and upper arms.
5. Tense all the muscles of your head, face, throat, and shoulders, including the forehead, cheeks, nose, eyes, jaw, lips, tongue, and neck.
6. Release all the tension in your head, face, throat, and shoulders.
7. Tense all the muscles in your chest, stomach, and lower back.
8. Release all the tension in your chest, stomach, and lower back.
9. Tense all the muscles in your thighs, buttocks, calves, and feet.
10. Release all the tension in your thighs, buttocks, calves, and feet.

Taking a Trip in Your Mind's Eye

1. Find a comfortable, quiet spot and assume a relaxed position.
2. Close your eyes.
3. Let your breathing begin to move lower in your body, moving toward your abdominal area. Each time you exhale, your breathing moves lower in your body toward your abdominal area.
4. Take yourself on a trip in your mind's eye to a place that is comfortable and relaxing, somewhere you have been or somewhere you would like to be. See all the sights associated with your quiet, relaxing place. Hear all the sounds associated with your quiet, relaxing place. Smell all the smells associated with your quiet, relaxing place. Taste any tastes associated with your quiet, relaxing place. Fully experience all the sensations associated with your quiet, relaxing place.
5. Totally immerse yourself in your quiet, relaxing place until you are ready to return, then gradually return from your trip, keeping the relaxation and calmness with you for as long as you wish. Then gradually open your eyes and resume your day.

Quick, Total Relaxing Exercise

1. Find a door with a strong door knob. Close the door tightly and grasp the door knob.
2. Place your feet shoulder distance apart, 2 to 3 feet from the doorknob, depending on the length of your body; the distance should be adequate to allow you to totally stretch out but not strain your body.
3. Let your body totally relax, and let your head drop toward your chest.
4. Hold this position until you feel your body relaxing; stand up, take a few deep breaths, and repeat steps 2–4.

Note: Relaxation tapes may be needed to learn the process since it is difficult to read while trying to learn to relax. They can be purchased at many bookstores or personally developed.

REFERENCES

Clark CC. (1996). *Wellness Practitioner: Concepts, Research, and Strategies.* New York: Springer Publishing Company.

Coldwell SE, Getz T, Milgrom P, Prall CW, Spadafora A, & Ramsay DS. (1998). CARL: A LABVIEW 3 computer program for conducting exposure therapy for the treatment of dental injection fear. *Behav Res Ther* 36(4):429–441.

Davis M, McKay M, & Eshelman E. (1995). *The Relaxation and Stress Reduction Workbook*. Oakland, CA: New Harbinger.

Epstein G. (1989). *Healing Visualizations Creating Health through Imagery*. New York: Bantam Books.

Penava SJ, Otto MW, Maki KM, & Pollack MH. (1998). Rate of improvement during cognitive-behavioral group treatment for panic disorder. *Behav Res Ther* 36(7–8):665–673.

Russo MB, Brooks FR, Fontenot J, Dopler BM, Neely ET, & Halliday AM. (1998). Conversion disorder presenting as multiple sclerosis. *Mil Med* 163(10):709–710.

Sharma VK, Narkiewicz K, Borys B, Furmanski J, Majkowicz M, & Krupa-Wojciechowska B. (1998). No title available. *Pol Merkuriusz Lek* 4(24):313–322.

Timmerman IG, Emmelkamp PNM, & Sanderman R. (1998). The effects of a stress-management training program in individuals at risk in the community at large. *Behav Res Ther* 36(9):863–875.

24

REFUTING IRRATIONAL IDEAS

Human beings engage in self-talk, an internal thought language, almost every moment of conscious life (Davis, Eshelman, & McKay, 1995). When self-talk is helpful and rational, all goes well. When self-talk is irrational and untrue, people experience stress and emotional disturbance, including depression.

The theory underlying refuting irrational ideas is that self-talk creates emotions. Anxiety, anger, and depression are created by unrealistic thoughts that are under the direct control of the individual (Ellis, 1980). Thirty years ago Rimm and Litvak (1969) found that negative self-talk produces significant physiological arousal, including tense muscles and other signs of stress.

At the root of irrational self-talk is the idea that things are being done to the individual. "She made me do it," "He makes me angry," "High places scare me." Two particularly damaging forms of self-talk are those that awfulize (e.g., a momentary pain is a sign of cancer or a heart attack), or absolutize (should, must, ought, always, and never are used to judge self or others' behavior). Both make situations more stressful and can blow a small incident into gigantic proportions.

Some common irrational ideas and their rational counterparts (Ellis, 1980; Davis et al., 1995) appear in Table 24.1.

Steps to Helping Clients Refute Irrational Ideas

Possibly as between-session homework, ask clients to:

1. Write down the facts of an event.
2. Write down any self-talk about the event.
3. Make a clear one or two word label (e.g., angry, depressed, fearful, anxious/ nervous, worthless) that describes their emotions regarding the event.
4. Refute the irrational self-talk identified in #2 by:

Table 24.1   Irrational Ideas and Their Rational Counterparts

Irrational Ideas	Rational Counterparts
I must have love.	It would be nice to have love, but I can survive without it.
Everyone must approve of me at all times.	It is impossible to have everyone like and approve of me at all times.
I must be competent at all times.	I am human; humans make mistakes, therefore I sometimes make mistakes, but they're fixable.
Some people are evil.	Some people act inappropriately and it would be better if they learned to change their behavior.
This situation is horrible; I can't stand it.	This situation might be inconvenient or painful, but I can handle it.
The unknown is something I need to fear.	The unknown can be novel and exciting.
It's easier to avoid responsibility than face it.	Adults have responsibilities to face.
I need something greater than me to rely on.	I have good judgment.
I'm a victim of my past.	I can identify old patterns and start changing them right now.
I'm helpless in this situation.	I can control how I interpret and emotionally respond to this situation.
People are fragile and need to be protected.	I can communicate my feelings openly directly.
Good relationships are based on self-sacrifice.	If I continue to deny my feelings and needs, I will feel bitter and withdrawn.
I must always please others or be abandoned or disapproved of.	People may not always agree with what I say or do, but I'm ready to take the consequences of my actions.
I have to be with other people to be happy.	Being alone is a growth-promoting experience.
There is a perfect love relationship for me.	No relationship is perfect.
I shouldn't have to feel pain.	Pain is an inevitable part of life.
My worth depends on what I achieve or produce.	My worth depends on my capacity to be fully alive, feeling all my feelings.
Anger is bad and destructive.	Anger is an honest communication that can be cleansing.
It is wrong to be selfish.	I am the best judge of what is right for me.
This situation is making me upset.	The situation is not doing anything to me.
Things should be better.	Things are exactly as they should be.
People pick fights with me.	It takes two people to have a conflict.
If I could find out the reasons for what's bothering me, I'd feel better.	The original cause of feelings is often lost in antiquity.

a. Selecting the irrational idea (see Ellis' listing of irrational ideas on page 217).

b. Asking if there is any rational support for the idea (there is no rational support for irrational ideas).

c. Finding any evidence that exists for the falseness of the idea (see Table 24.2).

Table 24.2   Refuting Irrational Ideas: Client Example

1. Write down an event that upset you: *My husband died.*
2. Write down your thoughts about what happened: *I can't believe this has happened to me. We were so happy together. I don't think I'm going to be able to live without him. Why is this happening to me? I must have done something to deserve it.*
3. Pick out the irrational ideas: *I can't believe this is happening to me. I don't think I'm going to be able to live without him. Why is this happening to me? I must have done something to deserve it.*
4. Write down the way you feel when you say the irrational ideas in number 3 above: *even more depressed and sad.*
5. Dispute and challenge your irrational ideas:

    a. Select one irrational idea: *I must have done something to deserve it.*
    b. Is there any rational support for this idea? *No.*
    c. What evidence exists for the falseness of your idea? *I've always been loving and faithful. I didn't do anything to cause his death.*
    d. Does any evidence exist for the truth of your idea? *No. I guess I just feel so miserable, I've talked myself into believing I must have had something to do with his death.*
    e. What is the worst thing that could happen to me? *I could go on feeling sad and blaming myself for his death.*
    f. What good things might occur? *I might realize that we had a wonderful life together, but that I can go on enjoying my life even though Ed isn't here anymore.*

6. Alternative self-talk: *I'm going to be OK. I can be alone and learn to enjoy it. I have inner strength.*
7. How I feel after my new self-talk: *I feel more peaceful. I know I have a lot of anger to release, but I see light at the end of the tunnel.*

d. Asking what evidence exists for the truth of the idea (irrational self-talk is the basis of unhappiness).

e. Asking: What is the worst thing that could happen to me if what I want doesn't happen? (Some ideas: I could feel inconvenience; I might have to accept the consequences of failure; I might be rejected as incompetent; I might feel more stressed; I might be deprived of various pleasures while dealing with the problem).

　　f. Asking: What good things might occur if what I want doesn't happen? (Some ideas: I might learn to tolerate frustration (pain, disapproval, etc.) better; I might improve my ability to cope with situations; I might become a more responsible person).

5. Substitute positive self-talk (Some ideas: Facing my problems is more useful than resenting it or running away; If I don't think negative thoughts I'll feel better; I can accept painful situations).

Client Form for Refuting Irrational Ideas

Provide the Client Form for Refuting Irrational Ideas to clients who are anxious, depressed, or angry. An example using the form is presented as well as the blank form for use with clients. See Tables 24.2 and 24.3 below. It is suggested that you also provide a copy of Table 24.1 above as an assist in identifying irrational and rational ideas.

Table 24.3　Refuting Irrational Ideas: Client Homework Sheet

1. Write down an event that upset you:
2. Write down your thoughts about what happened:
3. Pick out the irrational ideas:
4. Write down the way you feel when you say the irrational ideas in number 3 above:
5. Dispute and challenge your irrational ideas:

　　a.　Select one irrational idea:
　　b.　Is there any rational support for this idea?
　　c.　What evidence exists for the falseness of your idea?
　　d.　Does any evidence exist for the truth of your idea?
　　e.　What is the worst thing that could happen to me?
　　f.　What good things might occur?

6. Alternative self-talk:
7. How I feel after my new self-talk:

REFERENCES

Davis M, Eshelman ER, & McKay M. (1995). *The Relaxation & Stress Reduction Workbook.* Oakland, CA: New Harbinger.

Ellis A. (1980). *Growth Through Reason.* Palo Alto, CA: Science and Behavior Books.

Rimm DC, & Litvak SB. (1969). Self-verbalization and emotional arousal. *Journal of Abnormal Psychology* 74:181–187.

25

TOUCH THERAPIES

Touch is one of the major reasons people seek complementary therapists. This chapter explores the vast arena of touch, including Therapeutic Touch, massage, acupressure, and reflexology.

THERAPEUTIC TOUCH

Dolores Krieger, R.N. Ph.D., theorizes that *prana* (Sanskrit term for energy) is transferred in the healing act. She draws upon Eastern literature, finding apt analogies in Western thought. For example, the source of prana in Eastern thinking is the sun; likewise, the source of energy for photosynthesis is the sun. Eastern thinking contends that well people have an excess of prana; Western physiology texts state there is a great deal of redundancy in the human body. Krieger pictures the healer as a person with excess prana or energy who has a strong sense of commitment and intention to help people. Healing is described as "the conscious full engagement of your energies in the interest of helping another" (Krieger, 1993, pp. 17–18). Healers do not become depleted of energy because they are in a constant state of energy input-throughput-output. Healers become depleted of energy only if they become too closely identified with the process or try to draw on their own energy (rather than being a channel for energy).

A body of research is accumulating to back up the usefulness of therapeutic touch for anxiety (Heidt, 1979; Quinn, 1982; Hale, 1986), stress reduction (Kramer, 1990), pain (Meehan, 1985), and wound healing (Wirth, 1990).

According to Krieger, Therapeutic Touch works well with all stress-related diseases, having a significant effect on the autonomic nervous system, thereby influencing nausea, dyspnea, tachycardia, pallor, and peristalsis. Her report of one day's work at a clinic included seeing people with the following diagnoses: low back and shoulder pain, rheumatoid arthritis, post-abdominal surgery, cancer of the uterus, cancer of the breast, panic attack, TMJ, HIV/AIDS, multiple sclerosis, and peptic ulcer (Krieger, 1993, pp. 136–137). Therapeutic Touch has also been used during birth and delivery for post-episiotomy or cesarean healing, for colic, PMS, irritability, fatigue, elevated temperature, vomiting, diarrhea,

AIDS symptoms, chemotherapy, radiation sickness, and the dying process (Krieger, 1993, pp. 136–164.)

Signs that Therapeutic Touch has occurred in the client include a deepening of voice level; slowing and deepening of respirations; a sigh, deepened breathing, or comments such as "I feel relaxed"; peripheral flush or pinking of the skin due to dilation of peripheral blood vessels, first noticed in the face.

The healer centers and uses the hands (placed 2–3 inches from the client's skin) to move quickly over the body, reading signals of congestion or blockage of energy flow. The feeling of pressure sensed in the hands when congestion or blockage is present can be explained biophysically; as the healer moves the hands over the body, positive ions are picked up; this pressure sensation is related to atoms that have lost an electron. Positive ions are associated with feelings of lethargy, headache, irritability, and inflammations of the mucosal tissues; negative ions have been noted in areas that may induce a feeling of well-being, such as waterfalls and mountains (Robinson & Dirnfeld, 1967).

Krieger refers to the pressure as a "ruffling in the field"; the healer can remove the positive ions by shaking or wiping the hands. When the healer's hands are placed in the area of a "ruffle" and then the hands are moved away from the body in a sweeping gesture, the pressure is reduced and the feeling of energy flow is sensed; this is called "*unruffling the field*" (1979, p. 54). The unruffling motion can be used to soothe babies or reduce pain and tension. A 2- to 3-minute treatment is sufficient for children or the debilitated. With others the healer stops when the body feels balanced.

The object of Therapeutic Touch is to balance the healee's "field" so that symmetry of energy flow is restored. With practice the hands begin to move toward areas of unbalanced energy flow as they become more sensitive to changes in the field of another person's body.

Krieger reports that prana can be transferred to objects, especially cotton. By holding a piece of cotton in one hand and placing the other hand above the cotton and imagining reaching down to the hand under the cotton, energy can be transferred. In this way energy can be stored to be used at a later date when less energized or to prepare for clients' use when they feel fatigued (Krieger, 1979, pp. 28–29).

Therapeutic Touch Assessments

Krieger suggests that both telereceptive and personal field assessments be completed by the practitioner (1979, pp. 23–51). Prior to approaching a client, the practitioner centers to ensure a fully integrated, unified, focused assessment. Centering also protects the practitioner from picking up negative energy from the client and/or bringing his or her negative energy into the assessment process. Although Krieger does not suggest it, the practitioner can use imagery to place a shield of light (or some other substance) around the practitioner that allows energy to be picked up and sensed, but not to personally affect the practitioner.

Telereceptive assessments include:

- What do clients' voices tell me about their emotional level?
- What do clients' gaits tell me about their locomotion, guarding of body parts, hesitancy, tension level?
- What do clients' facial expressions tell me about their level of involvement with me?

Human field assessments are completed standing, facing clients, moving from the head quickly to the feet while holding the hands 2–3 inches away from their bodies. The back of the body is assessed while standing behind clients and moving in the same manner over the area until an assessment is completed. The practitioner does not hesitate in a spot, but continues moving the hands; if sensations are unclear, the practitioner moves body and hands to the side or away from clients and repeats the downward movement until an assessment is clear. The practitioner searches for differences in energy flow and uses the following questions to assess blocks:

- What does the area around clients tell me about them?
- Which areas of the body "feel" hot, cold, like shocks, pressure, tingling, pulsating, or dead to me?
- What sensations can be picked up on my hands on the right side of the body vs. the left, top vs. bottom, and back vs. front?

Clients can also be assessed while they are sitting in a chair or on the floor. The practitioner stands, kneels, or sits, depending on which position allows for the most complete assessment of the client.

In preparing to assess a client, the practitioner first enhances hand sensitivity by rubbing the palms together and gradually separating them until energy flow between the hands is noted. By experimenting, the distance between the two palms at which sensations are most evident is probably the distance from the client's body at which the practitioner's hands should be placed during assessment.

Therapeutic Touch Interventions

Prior to any intervention, the practitioner centers and holds the intention to heal. This is accomplished by placing the hands "with palms facing away from the body at the area where you felt the pressure and then move the hands away from the body in a sweeping gesture . . . " (Krieger, 1979, p. 54). Energy can also be directed from a higher energy area to a low energy area by moving the hands in the appropriate direction in a brushing movement.

Another use of therapeutic touch is to act as a channel for energy to bring it to the client from a universal energy source. This is particularly helpful if the client is fatigued or needs concentrated energy to heal. In this case, the practitioner centers, protects herself or himself, and pictures an energy source such as the sun, God, or another light or energy source. With eyes closed, the universal source of energy can be pictured being channeled through the practitioner's hands to the area in need of healing or energizing. For further information, see Krieger, D., *The Therapeutic Touch*, Englewood Cliffs, NJ: Prentice-Hall, Inc., 1979, or *Accepting Your Power to Heal, the Personal Practice of Therapeutic Touch*, Santa Fe, NM, 1993.

Therapeutic Touch Research Base

There have been numerous studies of therapeutic touch since the 1970s; results have been mixed, often due to the research design. More recent studies have used randomized designs.

Although there is some controversy over the conceptual base and exactly how Therapeutic Touch works, some research on the procedure has produced significant positive results. Snyder and colleagues (1995) found Therapeutic Touch helpful in reducing agitation behaviors in individuals with dementia. Wirth (1990, 1993) showed Therapeutic Touch helps in healing dermal wounds, accelerating healing in the treatment group.

A single-blinded randomized study of Therapeutic Touch for osteoarthritis of the knee in 25 individuals found significant improvement in function and pain for participants receiving treatment (Gordon, Merenstein, D'Amico, & Hudgens, 1998).

Turner and colleagues (1998) examined the effect of Therapeutic Touch on pain and anxiety in burn patients. Participants who received Therapeutic Touch in their study reported significantly greater reduction in pain and anxiety than those who received a sham version of the treatment.

Ireland (1998) studied the effect of Therapeutic Touch on the anxiety levels of HIV-infected children. She found that Therapeutic Touch resulted in lower overall mean anxiety scores, whereas the mimic Therapeutic Touch did not.

Uses

Therapeutic Touch has been used in the following situations:

1. To provide additional energy in the recuperative and self-healing processes of the client.
2. To aid in the relaxation response and reduce anxiety.
3. To relieve pain.
4. To accelerate healing.
5. To alleviate symptoms, including: dyspnea, coughing, hiccups, diarrhea, cramping abdominal pain, constipation, and fever (Snyder, 1998).

Precautions

Generally, clients will use the amount of energy needed and then will stop drawing energy; however, certain populations, including infants, children, elderly, and very ill adults may be very sensitive to treatments. In these cases, a 5-minute treatment with only gentle energy input is suggested. The head is also very sensitive and only cooling, sweeping movements are used.

Although it is possible to learn Therapeutic Touch in a seven-hour workshop, knowing when and how to use the procedure requires additional practice and a mentorship of several years to perfect the approach.

MASSAGE

Touch is one of the major reasons people seek complementary therapists. Massage is an easy, everyday skill that can be learned by almost anyone. There are some cultures where massage is taught to children the same way we teach ours to brush their teeth (Harrold, 1992, p. 7).

Massage is the oldest known healing art. The Orientals were using massage at least three thousand years before the birth of Christ. In China, it was one of the four classical forms of medical treatment, along with acupuncture, moxabustion (heat energy), and herbalism. In the East, massage remains an integral part of family life (Harrold, 1992, p. 8).

The effects of massage are psychological, mechanical, physiological, and reflexive. Massage is an art (a unique way of communicating without words and showing caring) and a science; systematic manipulation of the body tissue produces beneficial effects on the nervous and muscular systems, local and general circulation, the skin, viscera, and metabolism (Knaster, 1984, p. 247).

During massage, "the hands stimulate the sensory receptors of the skin and subcutaneous tissues, causing a series of reflex effects . . . some of these effects are capillary vasodilation or constriction, relaxation or stimulation of voluntary muscle contraction, and possible sedation or stimulation of pain in an area remote from the area being touched" (Tappan, 1984, p. 262).

Ruth Rice (1975), a wellness practitioner/psychologist and specialist in early child development, has researched sensorimotor stimulation of premature infants. She developed a specific stroking and massage technique. Her research demonstrated that touching, movement, and sound stimulate the nerve pathways and increase myelination (speeding up neurological growth), increase the release of the growth hormone somatrophin (leading to faster weight gain), and increase the output of the hypothalamus (general arousal center) leading to increased cell activity and endocrine functioning.

Massage Assessments

An assessment for the use of massage includes a determination of whether the following conditions or needs exist that are believed to be responsive to the approach:

- parent/infant bonding
- muscle spasm/soreness
- headache
- buildup of toxins and wastes
- inadequate healing
- fatigue
- tension
- premature infant development

Massage Interventions

Mechanical pressure is used in massage to:

> . . . rid the muscles of toxic products by "milking" these acids into the lymphatic and venous flow toward the heart. As the muscles relax, fresh blood flows into them, bringing necessary nutrition to the area. It is obvious that massage should *not* be given if there is a possibility of spreading inflammation; or of dislodging a thrombus, thus causing embolism; or if there is such obstruction that the mechanical assistance of massage could not improve the blood flow. However, massage given *first* to the proximal aspects of an injured limb will ensure that these circulatory pathways are open enough to carry the venous flow along toward the heart. (Tappan, 1984, p. 260)

There are five basic massage strokes.

1. *Effleurage* is the stroke that glides over the skin on the surface. It is the most common stroke. Effleurage is often used to begin a massage to explore for areas of tenderness or tightness. The hand is molded to the skin, stroking with firm and even pressure, usually upward.

2. *Petrissage* strokes lift the muscle mass and wring or squeeze it gently. Kneading manipulations are completed with the hands or fingers pressing and rolling the muscles. It stimulates muscular and nervous tissue, frees adhesions, and stretches adipose tissue to release toxins, pesticides, and additives stored there.

3. *Friction* with the heel of the hands, thumb, or fingertips (according to the area to be covered) penetrates into deeper tissue. The tissue under the skin is moved, not the fingers on the skin. The stroke is used to massage deep into joint spaces or around bony prominences, and can break down adhesions; it cannot affect a deep abdominal fibrositis, however.

4. *Vibration* is a fine, tremulous movement, sometimes only fluttering above a body part. It is used for its soothing effect which can also be accomplished via an electrical vibrator.

5. *Tapotement* is the use of the fists, or cupped palms, or the loose flinging of the hands to percuss a body area. The movement is done parallel to the muscle fibers to prevent trauma or spasm. This stroke is especially effective on tight shoulders or necks.

Experiment with a peer, friend, or family member with the various strokes and their effects prior to working with a client.

When practicing massage, it is wise to communicate with the client, asking where tense or tight spots are, experimenting with different strokes and asking for client input, and teaching the client self-massage measures. A massage is not a good time for general conversation, but practitioner and client should be focused on the massage experience. It is not unusual for clients to experience strong positive or negative feelings during massage; the body work releases unresolved feelings. If this should occur, stop the massage and use listening skills until the feelings and thoughts have been expressed. Resume when the client is ready.

There is little agreement about oil use; some practitioners recommend it for its reduction of friction; vegetable (not mineral) oil is suggested because it is easily absorbed by the skin, whereas mineral oil tends to clog the pores. Practitioners who do not recommend the use of any oil believe oil interferes with energy exchange and finger sensitivity.

The best surfaces for giving a massage are: a massage table, a water bed, the floor. Most beds are too soft to offer the support needed to apply the appropriate amount of pressure. When giving a massage on the floor, it will of necessity be shorter in duration to prevent damage to the practitioner. To counter some of the fatigue and stress, use foam knee padding or several sleeping bags to kneel on. A single mattress taken from a bed and placed directly on the floor will work, but its height is inconvenient. Working outside on the grass is a beautiful, serene experience for practitioner and client. A massage is best received in the nude, but if the client is uncomfortable, negotiate this item.

The practitioner's hands should be clean and fingernails trimmed down so the fingerpads are available for massage. Warm them if cold; either use warm water or rub them together vigorously. Be sure the client removes all jewelry, contact lenses, glasses, etc. The practitioner removes wristwatch, rings, and anything that will detract from the massage for the client.

Approach the client's body slowly, gradually working up to stronger strokes. Always keep at least one hand on the client; stopping and starting touch is disruptive to the flow of massage. Use body weight rather than hand and arm muscle to apply pressure. Use good body mechanics, bending the knees and relaxing into massage movements; breathe regularly, avoid holding the breath. Massage is intense, hard work. Remember to keep yourself well by altering the procedure with gentler approaches such as Therapeutic Touch, Jin Shin Jyutsu, or reflexology.

Begin a massage by holding the palms lightly against the client's forehead for a few moments, applying no pressure. Center and then begin massage. Table 25.1 gives information concerning massage.

Schneider (1979) advocates the use of *infant massage* as a relaxation and *bonding* procedure.

The most important elements that form the bond between mother and child include skin-to-skin contact, prolonged and steady eye-to-eye contact, and the soothing

Table 25.1 Massage

1. Ask the client to lie down on his or her back. Stand, sit, or kneel in back of the client's head. Massage the forehead with the balls of the thumbs ending at the temples.
2. Use the tips of the forefingers to press against the bony rims of the eye sockets.
3. Massage the chin between the thumb and forefinger.
4. Use the palms to massage both sides of the face.
5. Bring both hands under the neck (be careful of the ears); hold the head firmly and straight out from the neck. Knead the neck with one hand with the other hand moving from the bottom of the neck to the nape. Cradle the head firmly in your hands and pull out with a moderate pressure, hold the head, and begin making a cloverleaf (see Figure 25.1).

   This is an integrating brain movement that also releases tension. As you work, watch the client's chest for breathing changes; note skin color and sighs indicating relaxation. After completing the butterfly pattern, hold the head cradled in the hands for several practitioner and client breaths. Slowly place the client's head on the work surface and slowly move hands to the shoulders.
6. Push down on both shoulders with moderate to heavy pressure using body weight; hold the shoulders down through several slow breaths and then release the push, but keep the hands on the shoulders. Press in on the trapezius shoulder muscles looking for tight, hard, sore spots and lumps (muscle knots). When any is found, very gradually apply pressure with the ball of the thumb until reaching a point where it is sore; ask the client to tell you "when it's sore." Stop increasing the pressure at that point and hold the pressure you have. Wait for the client to relax; this can be enhanced by asking him or her to "breathe into my finger." Observe for signs of relaxation (muscle loosens, breath deepens and moves lower in the body) and then increase pressure with the ball of the thumb until another sore layer is reached. Repeat above. Move to locate and relax other sore areas in the shoulders.
7. Place the fingertips under the shoulders and move down to the shoulder blades, moving slowly if resistance is encountered, allowing the client to breathe in and out prior to moving the hands down. Watch for change in breathing and an opening up of the chest. When noted, go to number 8.
8. Place one hand on each side of the neck; turn the head to the left and to the right until resistance is met. If the neck is extremely tight, ask the client to "breathe into my hands" and gradually work the neck to the right and then to the left.
9. Holding the upper, back part of the head in both hands, lift the head as far forward as is comfortable. Stop when resistance is met, then gently nudge the head an inch farther forward. Slowly return the head to flat again.
10. Place the heel of the hands on the upper chest and push down and hold through several of the client's breaths, then release.
11. Place the hands under the client's armpits and gradually and firmly pull back and hold through several client breaths, then release.
12. Make fists of the hands and start at the middle of the chest below the collar bone and slide the knuckles out and down the torso following the ribs. Do successive movements until the entire rib cage has been covered. Avoid the abdominal area. Go lightly.

(continued)

Table 25.1   *(continued)*

13. Move to the right side of the client and make a firm, circular motion several times, radiating out from the navel and down toward the bladder. Knead the abdominal area.

14. Grasp the client's right arm with both hands; pull the arm firmly and slowly toward the foot, keeping it in proper alignment with the shoulder; hold through several client breaths, then release.

15. Starting at the wrist, knead up the forearm and upper arm; glide the hands down to the wrist. Knead the hand and down each finger, pulling each finger out with firm, strong pressure (you will get some resistance and/or hear a crack as pressure is released).

16. Repeat no. 14 and no. 15 with the other arm and hand.

17. Move to the client's feet. Grasp the right ankle with both hands and exert firm, even pressure by leaning back; this will release tension in the hip joint. Knead up from the ankle to the hip. Glide the hands down to the ankle.

18. Make a fist with the right hand and make circles on the bottom of the foot. Knead the rest of the foot and pull out firmly on each toe.

19. Complete no. 17 and no. 18 on the left leg and foot.

20. Ask the client to turn over on the stomach. Use pillows to support the abdomen, neck, etc. Knead up the back of the right leg. Grasp both ankles with the hands, lean back, and hold for one or two breaths, releasing any additional tension in the hip.

21. Knead up the back of the other leg.

22. Move to face the client's head. Using the weight of your body, push the client's shoulders down, hold through several client breaths, release.

23. Move to the right side of the client. Drum the outer edges of the hands lightly, but rapidly across the right shoulder and back several times. Drum down the spine and the leg and up the other leg to the top of the spine, down the spine and down the other leg, and back up to the top of the spine.

24. Place the heel of the right hand at the middle of the right shoulder and the heel of the left on the middle of the left buttock; alternately rock the body, pushing down first with the right heel (hand) and then with the left heel (hand). Complete this rocking motion 2–3 times. Then place the heel of the left hand in the middle of the left shoulder and the heel of the right hand in the middle of the right buttock; rock 2–3 times, remembering to breathe and bend (see Figure 25.2).

25. Place the right hand underneath the lower abdomen and the left hand directly above on the lower back; push up with three fingers with the right hand and work down all five meridians (see Figure 25.2).

26. Right (or lower hand) pushes on the coccyx (sitbone) toward head; upper hand works from the spine outward, working one vertebra at a time (see Figure 25.2).

27. Find coccyx, then go 2″ out to the right from it; client will feel some pain/pressure; when area has been located, release the pressure and work on the left shoulder and neck area with the other hand (keep the hand in place on the coccyx). Repeat, reversing hands and moving 2″ out to the left from the coccyx (see Figure 25.2).

28. Stand on the left side of the client, left hand to the left of the cervical spine, right hand just below it; work down the side of the spine with fingertips of both hands, making two clockwise circles into each spinal process; this soothes. Work around the coccyx and up the other side of the spine making two counterclockwise circles, up and into the spinal processes; this stimulates.

Table 25.1 *(continued)*

29. Place the hands on the client's head and quickly run both hands down the head, shoulders, arms, legs, and off the end of the feet. Return to the head and repeat until the entire back of the body has been covered with this quick, light movement.
30. Ask the client to slowly turn over when ready. Place the hands lightly on the client's cheeks and hold for a minute or two.
31. Move to the right side of the client, facing his or her head, and repeat the quick movement of the hands from the head down and off the body until every spot on the body has been covered.
32. Let the client rest for a few minutes while you meditate or close your eyes and relax.

Note: If, during massage, any muscle knots are found, use deep, hard pressure with the thumb; if that does not release the muscle, use acupressure, pushing straight in with the thumb for 8–10 seconds, release, and repeat until muscle relaxes. Additionally, ask the client to picture that muscle relaxing. For further information, see: Downing, G., *The Massage Book,* New York: Random House, 1972, or D. Baloti Lawrence, *Massage Techniques,* New York: Perigee, 1986.

high pitched sounds of mother's voice in response to her infant's cry. Infant massage which serves as communication between parent and infant helps cement that bond. Baby learns to enjoy the wonderful comfort and security of loving and being loved. She acquires knowledge about her own body, as mother shows her how to relax a tense arm or back, or helps her release some painful gas. (p. 17)

Fathers are encouraged to learn infant massage. It is an excellent tool, providing quality experience for father and infant. The infant learns father can touch gently and lovingly and can be counted on to satisfy physical and emotional needs. The father learns to satisfy his infant and enhance his self-esteem and self-confidence.

Schneider (1979, p. 25) suggests the first 9 months are the ideal time to start. Daily massages up to 6 or 7 months of age are recommended. As the child becomes more active, once or twice a week is sufficient, but "growing pains" can be reduced through a pre-bedtime massage. Children who are not introduced to massage until age 3 or 4 can be offered a brief, gentle back massage at bedtime; in time, children begin asking for a massage. Older children can be taught to give their brothers and sisters a massage; this will increase bonding between the children, enhance the older child's self-esteem, and help the older child resolve being replaced when a new infant is born. Rolling, milking, and circular strokes can be used with the infant. The arms and legs can be kneaded just as in adult massage.

All babies will fuss and cry at some times during massage; this is expected. It may be that parts of their bodies they were not aware of are sore to the touch; a gentler massage in those areas will relax the infant. For the first 3 months of life, infants may resist having their arms massaged, since moving the arms so far from the body may seem unnatural; gentle shaking and patting movements are suggested in this case. Back massage is usually enjoyed at this time.

From 4 to 7 months, soreness and tension often moves to the back (crawling and sitting begins) and face (sucking and teething). At the end of the first year,

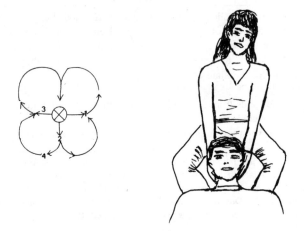

Figure 25.1   Integrating and relaxing the brain.
Sitting on the floor facing the back of the client's head, or standing behind the head of the massage table or bed, the practitioner exerts a slight, equal pull straight back with both hands from underneath the neck. Beginning and ending at midpoint **X**, the head is guided through two loops on the right side of midpoint and then two on the left side of midpoint. The head is gently placed on the floor, table, or bed, and hands are very slowly released from underneath the neck.

1a = rock
1b = rock
2 = work down meridians
3 = right or lower hand on coccyx/sitbone,
  other hand works up and outward from spine
4 = right or lower coccyx, left hand works
opposite shoulder and neck area

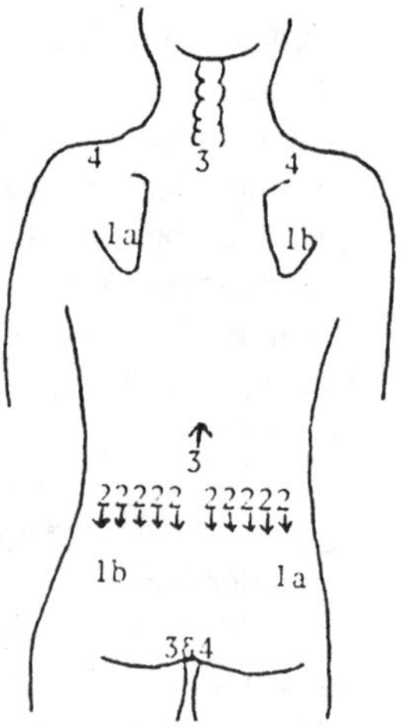

Figure 25.2   Back massage.

tension may move to the legs. Infants who have been massaged from infancy will help by massaging themselves and by one and a half years will massage their dolls and teddy bears, and often their mothers.

Schneider (1979, pp. 31, 76) suggests the following interventions when the infant fusses:

1. Breathe deeply and relax. Use affirmations including, "I now let go of tension. My body is relaxed. I now let go of thoughts. My mind is open and free. I am the gentle power of love, flowing through my hands to (baby's name)."
2. Stop in the middle of the massage to cuddle, hold, or walk the baby.
3. Give the baby a teether or small toy to play with or chew on.

Scientific Base

There is conflicting evidence regarding the use of massage, especially back massage (Corley, Ferriter, Zeh, & Gifford, 1995; Longworth, 1982; Meek, 1993). Massage has been shown to stimulate the body's ability to control pain naturally by producing endorphins and other pain-controlling chemicals (Ironson et al., 1996). It has also been used in a controlled study to help premature infants gain weight and be discharged sooner (Field et al., 1986), to increase natural killer cells (Groer et al., 1994), to reduce dermatitis symptoms in children (Schachner, Field, Hernandez-Reif, Duarte, & Krasnegor, 1998), decrease anxiety and stress hormone levels for individuals with fibromyalgia (Sunshine et al., 1996), and reduce depression in adolescent mothers (Field, Grizzle, Scafidi, & Schanberg, 1996).

Uses

Massage has been used in the following ways (Snyder & Cheng, 1998):

1. To promote relaxation (by decreasing aggressive behavior, lessening fatigue and pain, and producing sleep).
2. To improve mobility.
3. To decrease the need for an episiotomy.
4. To reduce edema.
5. To increase communication.
6. To lessen anxiety.
7. To lessen depression.
8. To increase well-being.

Precautions

Obtain the permission of the client before using massage. Not everyone reacts positively to being touched, especially by strangers. Avoid massage when the skin is broken, red, bruised, or has a rash or varicosities. Individuals with breathing problems, arthritis, and fresh from abdominal surgery may be unable to lie prone for a massage. Individuals with transmittable skin diseases, unhealed wounds, postoperative conditions, and blood clots are not considered good candidates for massage.

Individuals diagnosed with cancer should not be massaged (cancerous cells may break lose from the original source), nor should women who are pregnant (it could precipitate an abortion). Individuals with cardiac conditions may be safely massaged (Bauer & Dracup, 1987), but if there is chronic heart or kidney disease, caution should be used. Massage may not be appropriate for some cases of edema; it can encourage more swelling and bleeding. Individuals with nerve injury may find the skin pressure painful. Massage should not be applied to the abdomen of individuals with high blood pressure and peptic ulcer nor to burned areas until they are healed. Foot reflexology (a type of foot massage described later in this chapter) or Therapeutic Touch should be considered for all of these populations.

ACUPRESSURE

Acupressure is the predecessor of acupuncture. It grew from the instinctual response of massaging sore muscles by pressing sore spots on the body and noting the positive effects. Currently, the term is applied to a number of techniques of applying pressure to stimulate acupuncture points on the body.

Acupressure releases tension and relieves pain. It is a preventive treatment used to balance energy. Chinese medicine contends that the vital force, *chi*, that controls the functioning of the body systems permeates living tissue circulating along clearly defined pathways called meridians. There are 12 organ meridians; each one takes its name from the organ to which it is connected. Energy is believed to flow through each of the 12 meridians, flowing into one another, forming a continuous pathway for energy. When energy is blocked, it can be balanced by applying pressure to specific points.

Acupressure Assessments

An assessment for the use of acupressure includes identifying the existence of the following conditions or needs that have been found to respond to the technique:

- headache
- arthritis
- back tension and lower back pain
- menstrual discomfort
- labor and delivery
- morning sickness

- deficient lactation or mastitis
- overall balance
- appetite balance
- circulation balance
- digestion balance
- elimination balance
- fainting
- fracture healing
- inflammation
- motion balance
- muscle balance
- pain control
- sciatic relief
- substance abuse
- throat
- strains, sprains, and their prevention

Acupressure Interventions

The palms of the hands, the thumbs, or the four fingers apply 3–5 kg of pressure to the client's body for 3–5 seconds in acupressure. Pressure is gradually increased until the maximum pressure is reached; then it is decreased. The direction of pressure is toward the center of the client's body. The weight of the whole body, not just the hands, is used (Serizawa, 1972, pp. 24–25).

Nickel (1984) suggests preventive acupressure for sports activities. (See Figures 25.3, 25.4). Areas of common injury are focused on prior to engaging in

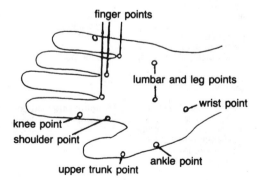

Figure 25.3   Prevention acupressure (increases circulation to the most commonly injured areas).

(Source: Nickel, 1984, pp. 24–73.)

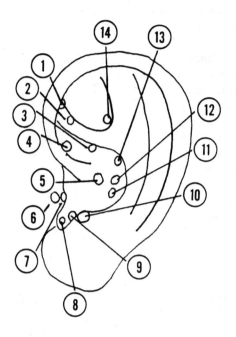

Figure 25.4 Overall balancing: ear acupressure.

Apply firm pressure with thumb ball and index finger for 1 minute, in 5-second-on and 5-second-off intervals. Use right ear.

(*Source:* Nickel, 1984, pp. 83–103.)

① **sympathetic point** (perspiration, stomach spasm, pain, coordination)

② **sciatic point** (sciatica)

③ **kidney point** (fractures, dizziness, ear ringing, edema, hearing loss, weariness, electrolyte imbalance, kidney injury)

④ **large intestine point** (constipation, diarrhea, hemorrhoids, respiration)

⑤ **stomach point** (indigestion, nausea, belching, heartburn, peptic ulcer, distension)

⑥ **hunger point** (under or overweight, anorexia, bulimia)

⑦ **adrenal point** (inflammation, swollen joints, muscles, tendons, allergies, cellulitis, common cold, fatigue, respiration, fever, frostbite, sinuses)

⑧ **steroid point** (allergies, inflammation, shock)

⑨ **ovary point** (painful menstruation, amenorrhea, infertility)

⑩ **occiput point** (jet lag, car and sea sickness, convulsions, lock jaw, stiff neck)

⑪ **spleen point** (abnormal uterine bleeding, indigestion, prolapsed viscera)

⑫ **relax muscles point** (liver, pain)

⑬ **liver point** (headaches, circulation, iron deficiency anemia, arthritis, muscle spasm, stomach gas, seizures)

⑭ **neurogate point** (body pain, allergies, anxiety, asthma, coughing, hypertension, insomnia, itching)

the activity, thus strengthening the body against injury during play. Nickel (1984) also suggests an overall balancing point using ear acupressure techniques; see Figure 25.4. The points suggested in the two illustrations can also be used once an injury is incurred; acupressure should not be used to avoid the pain associated with a strain, tear, or fracture in order to continue with vigorous exercise, but can be used in conjunction with other treatments.

Lowe and Nechas (1983) suggest specific acupressure points of relief of pain. The Hegu point is the key to relieving pain in the head, neck, and arms. To locate the point:

> . . . lay your left hand on a flat surface. Position the thumb so that it forms a right angle with the index finger. Now feel along the bone that extends back from the knuckle of the index finger. Along the index finger bone is the Hegu point. The point actually lies a little down and under the index finger bone. If you press down right alongside the bone, you have to press sideways, after you reach a sufficient depth, to reach a point under the bone. . . . As you press harder you should feel the pressure radiating along the nerves in your hand. This sensation signals that you are on the Hegu point. (p. 15)

Early morning stiff necks, dental pain, and headaches respond well to hard pressure on the Hegu point.

Another location for headache is the Fengchi points on the back of the head, in the depressions on either side of the cervical vertebrae below the occipital bone. Pushing hard up and into the skull will relieve some headaches. One or the other points, or a combination of Hegu and/or Fengchi works for most people; experimentation is necessary. Tenderness of a meridian point is the best indicator the point has been located.

A point that brings neckache relief is Xuehai, located on the inside of the thigh, just back of the knee cap. The Liangqui point is located on the outside of the thigh behind the knee cap. The Tiantu point can help asthma; it is at the base of the throat right above the suprasternal notch; pressing this point on children may cause a slight choking sensation that may frighten the child.

The Yuyao point in the middle of the eyebrow eases fatigue, and Taichong, at the place where the big and second toes meet, energizes. Zusanli, about 3″ below the knee, relieves abdominal pain and motion sickness as well as energizes. Yongquan, located just behind the ball of the foot, energizes and revives after a faint (Lowe & Nechas, 1983, pp. 1–29).

Patterson (1984) suggests the following acupressure points for specific problems: all points in Figure 25.5, Neck and Shoulder Release.

Jin Shin Jyutsu is a gentle form of acupressure which can be very effective. Three fingers of each hand—index, middle, and ring—are used to assess pulses indicating the flow of bodily energy. There are 26 specific points on the body used to treat specific symptoms. The practitioner (or client) first learns to assess the pulses, then to keep the fingers on that area until all three pulses in both hands flow evenly. Points are usually used in a certain pattern to achieve release or balance. Figure 25.6 shows the energy release points.

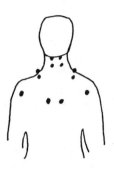

Figure 25.5   Acupressure for neck and shoulder release.

Pressure is increased until the client is comfortable with a firm amount. The pressure is held steadily until a very faint even pulse is felt at the acupoint. Clients can be taught to do their own acupressure; in this case, they can be taught to hold the pressure until the pulse is felt. It can take 3 to 10 minutes or even longer for severe problems. The release should be slow and easy and some pain may result as blocked areas open and trapped chemicals and flow release. There is no one correct pressure for individuals or acupoints; they can differ considerably. As for other complementary practices, it is important to converse with the client and observe for positive and negative responses to treatment. To work on hard to reach spots (such as backs), clients can be counseled to ask a partner to apply pressure or place a tennis ball on the floor and then lie on top of it.

Uses

Acupressure has been used for allergies, angina pectoris, arthritis, asthma, athletic injuries, back problems, chronic fatigue syndrome, common cold, constipation, diarrhea, earache, headache, immune problems, indigestion, insomnia, motion sickness, nausea, chronic pain, TMJ syndrome, and toothache. Studies have shown that acupressure can hasten recuperation from stroke and surgery, relieve morning sickness, indigestion, and backache of pregnancy, alleviate the pain of childbirth, and enhance recuperation (Ballegaard, Noorelunds, & Smith, 1996; Chow, 1998; Fan et al., 1997; Felhendler & Lisander, 1997; Somerville, 1997; Zeidenstein, 1998).

Precautions

Because significant pressure can be used in acupressure, caution should be exercised in its use. Never press on an open wound, swollen or inflamed skin, bruises,

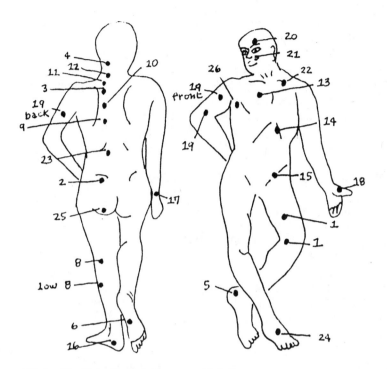

Figure 25.6   Jin Shin Jyutsu Pressure Points.
S = same side O = opposite side

Abdominal bloat: Hold 2 and O-High 1
Abdominal congestion: Hold 1 and O-26, then 1 and 8; then 13 and O-11 then
   23 and S-1 or high 1
Allergies: Hold 3 and S-15; then 10 and S-hi 19
Appetite: Hold 13 and O-11; 14 and S-19
Arms: Hold 3 and S-15; 11 and S-25; 12 and O-4
Arthritis: Hold 10 and S-3
Back, Low pain: Hold 2 and S-8; S-2 and O2; 4 and O-21
Balance (emotional/physiological): Hold 14 and S-19
Birth (pelvic opening): Hold hi 1s, 2s; 2s and O1s and O-8s
Bites (bug): 9s, left hand over right hand on bite
Bladder problems: Hold S-15s, S-2s, 2 and O-15; O1 and O-8
Bleeding: Left hand over right on top of bleeding
Bowels: S-15s; 2s; 2s and O8s; then O-1s
Brain: 4 and O-21; S-12 and 4; S-19, 21 and O-23; 22 and S-3
Breasts (lumps): S-10s; S-19s
Burns: Palms on top of burn, then place palms (with fingers pointing toward the
   head) on calves and hold for 20 minutes or more
Cancers: 15 and S-3; 16 and S-12; 17 and O-16; 18 and S-4; 19 and S-14; 23
   and S-1; 25 and S-11

Circulation: 13 and O-1; both hi 19s; 3 and S-15
Colds: 10s; 11s; 12s; 1s; 17s
Constipation: L18 and R11, then R2
Diabetes: 23s, 9s
Diarrhea: R8 and L11, then L2
Digestion: Hold both hi 1s (on self, cross hands); hi 19 and O-hi 1
Dizziness: pinch under nose hard; 8 and S11
Ears: 13s; S-12 and 4; 21 and O-23; 22 and S-3
Emphysema: 10 and S-hi 19; 13 and O-11; 15 and S-3
Energy, Lack: hi 19s; 2 and O-9; 23 and S-1; 25 and S-11
Eyes: 4s; 10s; 3s
   Twitching: Hold opposite eye, hold 4 and opposite 20,21, 22
Face, tension: 21s
Fat: 1s; hi 1s; 23s; 25s; hi 19s
Flatulence: 11 and S-25
Flu/Fever: 3 and S-15; 4 and O-21; 15 and S-3
Gout: 16 and S-8
Groin: 2 and S-1; 3 and S-15
Headache: 8s; 11s; 16s; 24s; hold big toes or thumbs
   Migraine: 20s; 21s; 4s; 7s; 16s; 10s; 9s; 4s
Heart, attack: 3s; 9s; 14s
Hemorrhoids: O-8 and O-1
Hip: S-11 and S-15
Hormone, imbalance: 2s; ring fingers; on self, hold 12s
Hyperactivity: 13s
Hypertension: 19s; 16s; 15s and 3s together
Hypoglycemia: 12s; 19s; 13s and 9s
Insomnia: 18s and thumbs, 16s; 17s; 18s; 19s
Jet lag: 25s; lock fingers or hold each finger
Joint pain: 19 and 3
Kidney: 23s; 5s; 6s
   Stones: 3s; 23s; 2s; 25 and hi 11s same side
Knees: 24s
Labor: 2s; hi 1s
Legs: 25 and center back of leg; 25s
   Charley horse: 25 and 12; then S-15 and S-7
   cramps: S-15 and toes; S-25 and 11
   fall asleep: 25s same side and O-1s
Leukemia: 9s; 26s
Lungs: 9s; 10s; 22s
Mastectomy: 5s; 6s; 7s; 8s; 16s; 17s; 18s; 19s
Menopause: 22s
Menstruation: 2 with O-8 and 1o 8 to 16; lo 8s and 15s
   ovulation distress: 1 and O-8
Motion sickness: 14s; 25s
Muscles, tension: 8s; 16s; 25s
Nausea: 14s; 18s

Nervous system: 17s
  nervousness: 11s
Newborn: 2 and O-9
Nightmares: 10 and S-hi 19
Nose: 3s; 4s; 11s
Overeating: Hold hi 1s (fingers pointing down)
Overweight: 21s; 23s; 25s
Pain: S-20s; right hand over left and cover pain area, 9 and 15 and hold 10 on
  opposite side of pain with same side 9, then 15
Paralysis: for left side, hand on right 8; for right side, hand on left 8
Parkinson's: 3 and S-15;10 and S-hi 19; 15 and S-3; 23 and S-1; 25 and S-11
PMS: 1 and O-26; 2 and O-9; 13 and O-11; 11 and S-19; 15 and S-3
Prostate: 23s
Sciatica: Hold left 11 as anchor, and L hand on L23, then L2 (for left pain use
  R pulse points)
Shingles: 9s
Shock: Thumbs on R temple, fingers on R 4; then Thumbs on L temple, fingers
  on L4
Shoulders: 3s; 19s (opposite side)
  To release: 8s; 1s; 16s
Sinuses: 4s and O-21
Snoring: 14 and S-19
Throat: 4s; 10s; 11s; 12s; 13s;
TMJ: 21s
Tonsils: 4 and O-16; then opposite lo 8
Varicose veins: 15 and S-13; 23 and S-1; 25 and S-11
Viruses: hold 3s and 11s together; then 9s; and 10s
Whiplash: 2s; 8s; 9s; 10s; 23s; 25s;
Yeast infection: 13s; 23s

Source: Extracted from *High Touch, Hands on Energy Workbook II,* Betsy Dayton, Edgewater,
Colorado: Betsy Dayton, 1984.

varicose veins, or a lump. Sites of recent surgery and suspected bone injury
should also be avoided. Direct pressure on the carotid artery should be avoided
with individuals suffering from atherosclerosis. Avoid pressure to the lower
abdomen on pregnant women and avoid using Spleen 6 or Large Intestine 4,
which may induce abortion (Somerville, 1997).

REFLEXOLOGY

Theory of Reflexology

Reflexology is based on the premise that body organs have corresponding reflex
points on other parts of the body. The reflex points are believed to be up to 20

times more sensitive than the corresponding organs. The foot is viewed as one of the scanner screens that records body functions. Working the reflexes in the feet helps rebalance organs that are functioning properly by releasing blocks that impede the smooth flow of body energy. Reflex points also influence functional relationships to that organ. For example, stimulating the heart reflex on the foot helps balance energy flow to the heart as well as the rest of the circulatory system (blood vessels, lymphatics, etc.). There are other areas with reflex points (wrist, hand, ear, neck, abdomen, face, head, arms, legs, nose, and iris), but the feet are the most effective because:

1. They link with energy from the earth and are strong energy poles of the body.
2. Working on feet is relatively nonthreatening and noninvasive.
3. Feet accumulate deposits of acids and tensions (due to the effect of gravity pressure, and the normal wear and tear of walking upright), causing tissue degeneration which can easily be felt, seen, and treated.
4. Touching the feet is a soothing gesture that can deeply affect others; for example, agitated children can be calmed by rubbing their feet.
5. Clearly charted representation of the body organs on the foot are available.
6. Because feet are usually covered with shoes and socks, they remain tender to the touch and more sensitive than some other reflex points. Additionally, there is less body musculature that might interfere with assessment and intervention than in most other parts of the body.
7. Feet are a symbolic representation of the infinite energy in the universe. Jesus washed the feet of his disciples, linking, cleansing, protecting, and blessing their whole being (Berkson, 1977, pp. 1–2).

Berkson has developed the Integrated Treatment from her study of reflexology, nutrition (she has a master's degree in the subject), acupressure (she is a certified shiatsu therapist), yoga, massage, and polarity. Her method combines diet, exercise, and healing visualization and affirmations to broach the physical, mental, spiritual, and artistic. Blocks are released and deposits are thrown off, increasing vitality of the whole person and increasing relaxation and activity potential (physical). The act of reflexology is a giving and receiving, a sharing of communication resulting in confidence and calming (mental). Together, healer and healee call upon the healing energy of the universe to surround, uplift, and permeate; the use of affirmations and the projection of a positive healing environment is a spiritual act of being of service to others (spiritual). The Integrated Treatment calls for knowledge, skills, and a personalized interaction between healer and healee to produce healing (art) (Berkson, 1977, pp. 7–8).

Reflexology Assessments

Figure 25.7 presents the foot reflexes used for assessment and treatment. Berkson (1977) suggests the following assessments be made:

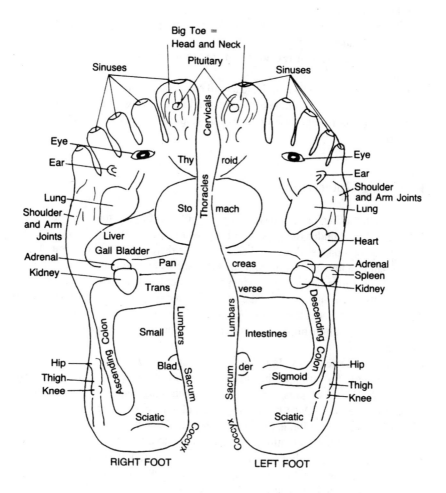

Figure 25.7   Foot reflexology points.

Sources: Extracted from *The Foot Book*, D. Berkson, New York: Harper & Row, 1977; *The Massage Book*, G. Downing, New York: Random House, 1972.

- What does the skin color tell me?
- Are the heels of the shoes worn evenly?
- Are the eyes clear?
- Is the tongue coated?
- Are the nails strong and the hair shiny?
- What do the client's voice and posture tell me?
- Which joints rotate easily?
- Which reflex points are the most tender or the most difficult to relieve?
- How does bone feel under the skin?

- How do muscles feel?
- What temperature differences are there? (an even, warm temperature indicates balance)
- What differences in texture are there? (bunions and callouses can indicate imbalances)
- What areas on the foot indicate a hard resistance? (indicating tension, deposits, or degeneration, unless a bone, tendon, or ligament resides there)
- What areas feel hollow or recessed? (indicating lack of nutrition and energy imbalance)

Reflexology Interventions

Prior to attempting reflexology, sensitivity of the fingers must be developed. Placing a thread under the page of a book is a good exercise. When that can be sensed, try two pages, three, and so on. Using different materials, dental floss, rubber bands, and seeds of different sizes also works. As with other body therapies, it is not wise to practice them when feeling depleted or ill oneself since it is possible to drain energy from the client. Protecting oneself, using energizing affirmations, and attending to other dimensions of wellness (nutrition, stress management, relationships, environment) will tend to make depletion an uncommon happening.

Pressure in reflexology should evoke a "good hurt" or pressure that is comfortably tolerated. To estimate the pressure needed, practice pressing a bathroom scale to 20–25 lb. of pressure. Very sore spots may require a buildup to this amount of pressure. Once the appropriate amount of pressure is found, hold it until a rhythmic pulsation is felt or until the client experiences a release (observe for change to a deeper breathing pattern, change to a better skin tone, relaxation in facial expression, and/or the client's words). For very painful spots, return to them again and again rather than trying to relieve the pain all at once; too much work all at once may bruise the capillaries.

Practice strengthening and using the *thumb*, for it is the most sensitive of the fingers. Continued experimentation with reflexology will strengthen them. As with other body work, working with the fingertips in reflexology promotes the practitioner's physiological balance; every time the foot is pressed, spinal and brain energy are activated in both practitioner and client (Berkson, 1977, p. 33).

Preparation for reflexology with a client:

1. Remove nail polish from fingernails and cut nails so nailpads are exposed. Shake, stretch, squeeze, and wash hands so they are relaxed and warm.
2. Find a quiet spot and ask the client to assume a comfortable sitting or lying position. Avoid music, disruptions, and any conversation except that related to the effects of the strokes.
3. Assume a relaxed position; a relaxation exercise can assist both practitioner and client to prepare for a reflexology session. Visualizing a protective

covering of light and affirming that no negative energy will be transferred from client to practitioner is a safety measure.

4. Ask the client to relax and let go and avoid trying to assist.
5. Hold the client's feet in the hands for a few minutes while centering to orient both to the physical contact. Remember to breathe throughout the session.
6. Begin with the right foot. Avoid removing the hands from the foot until all steps have been completed. Each petrissage stroke (releases toxins) should be followed by an effleurage stroke (encourages removal of toxins to the bloodstream).

   A. Take the foot in both hands and stretch the sole gently, toes toward ankle and toes toward sole several times; note callouses, bunions, degree of flexibility, etc.

   B. Hold the front of the foot in the left hand (reverse if left-handed) and the heel in the right hand; rotate the heel slowly and gently clockwise and then counterclockwise; note resistances and range of motion.

   C. Grab hold of the foot and wring it like a sponge, one hand above the other, twisting in opposite directions; continue up and down the foot from ankle to toes, using steady, firm pressure. In this movement as in many others, the tendency for novices is to be too gentle; a firm pressure is needed to counteract tickling and to obtain results.

   D. Stimulate the lymphatic drainage by pressing the lymphatic drainage point between the big and second toe (Figure 25.7). Use the thumb to stretch the skin from the heel along the outside of the foot to the toes using 20–25 lb. of pressure. Remember to breathe.

   E. Sandwich the foot in between the two hands; use the knuckles to rub over all points on the foot. Breathe.

   F. Start at the end of the big toe and use the thumbs to stretch the tendons toward the ankle up into the lymphatic area. Do all toes and the spaces in between. Breathe.

   G. Anchor the heel with one hand and push on the ball of the foot with the other palm to the client's limit; hold for 15–30 seconds, then release. Breathe.

   H. Anchor the heel with one hand and press the toes and foot toward the floor with the other to the client's limit and hold for 15–30 seconds, then release.

   I. Rotate the foot laterally and hold and then medially and hold. Rotate the whole foot clockwise and counterclockwise.

   J. Hold heel firmly in left hand and firmly press all inside and outside ankle reflexes for 3–5 seconds on each spot (see Figure 25.7). Rub ankle in an upward movement (effleurage).

   K. Stabilize the foot with one hand, using the other to grasp the big toe firmly with thumb on top and forefinger on the back; make stretching movements from the base to the top of the toe; repeat on each toe. Work each toe medially, laterally, forward, and back. Breathe.

L. Hold the big toe close to its base, thumb on top where it meets the foot and forefinger beneath the joint connecting the toe to the foot. Support the foot well with the other hand and pull the toe straight out to the toe's maximum stretch for 10 seconds, then use a firm jerk straight back, listening for a cracking sound; some toes will "crack," while others will not; avoid forcing it. Jerk once or twice on each toe and then move on to the next one; return later to release tension; this movement stimulates tendons and clears the head and neck of congestion since all meridians and nerve endings for the brain and neck are stimulated (Berkson, 1977, p. 47).

M. Begin with the big toe; hold each toe in succession firmly and work down its corresponding tendon toward the ankle.

N. Begin with the big toe and rotate each toe three times in a full circle clockwise and then counterclockwise; observe for resistance and gritty sounds (indicating crystal formation).

O. With the fingers on one hand on the top of the toes and the other hand anchoring the heel, push forward firmly, hold a stretch, go a bit further, then release (toe extension release).

P. Grasp the toes firmly with hand, thumb on top of toes downward while pushing up from underneath at the lung reflex; this movement will release tension in the shoulder girdle. Optional: flex and extend each toe individually.

Q. Hold the big toe firmly and pull it toward the other foot; smack the side of the thoracic reflex (bony ridge beneath the toes) with the top of the palm as if clapping the hands; repeat 8–10 times. Releases tight shoulder blades, clears the neck, throat, eye, and ear, and reduces bunions (Berkson, 1977, p. 49).

R. Press firmly on all points of the big toe, front, back, side, and top. Repeat with each toe using very firm thumb pressure. Stimulate the web of each toe with the thumb and forefinger, top and bottom; use a pinching movement. Effective for eyes, ears, and sinuses.

S. Inch along the top of all toes with fingernail and flick each toenail up and away from the toe. Nails store electromagnetic current; flicking and stimulating the periphery stimulates meridians and releases energy (Berkson, 1977, p. 52).

T. Stimulate the eye and ear points at the base of the toes and stretch the skin from the small toe to the inside of the big toe; this will drain the sinuses and soothe the eyes and ears (Berkson, 1977, p. 52).

U. Stimulate venous drainage by rubbing each toe from its tip to its base.

V. Start with the spinal points on the sole of the foot (Figure 25.7), working the sacral and lumbar area by the heel up to the cervical area by the big toe, then work down the other side to the heel; follow with friction and effleurage.

W. Press all points on the lateral, medial, and top of the foot and ankle using knuckles; follow with effleurage.

X. Use a wringing motion up the leg; push the middle three fingers under the tibia from the ankle to the knee. Observe for swelling, granular tissue, and deposits; work them out with rubbing and pressure.

Y. Support the leg and use the middle finger or knuckle to press up the center of the calf from the Achilles tendon to the knee, stimulating the endocrine glands; highly stressed clients are tender there (Berkson, 1977, p. 56).

Z. Push firmly all the way up the leg from the ankle to the thigh, increasing the lymphatic and blood flow. Close by clapping the foot from heel to toe, and then brushing the hands down the legs several times from the knee off the end of the toes and then several inches away from the body. Repeat A–Z with left foot.

Figure 25.7 can be used to treat specific conditions, e.g., pancreas for diabetes; small intestines area for digestive or assimilation difficulties; stomach for heartburn, nausea, bad breath, vomiting, or tightness under breastbone. Working on the toes will assist with headache, tension, congestion, sinus trouble, weak eye muscles, fatigue, etc. Although reflexology can be used this way, it is recommended the steps from A–Z be completed daily as a preventive measure. For further information, see: Berkson, D., *The Foot Book: Healing through Reflexology*, New York: Harper & Row, 1977; Ingham, E., *Stories the Feet Tell through Reflexology*, St. Petersburg: Ingham Publishing, 1984.

Scientific Base

Snyder and colleagues (1995) tested the amount of time for giving a hand massage. They found that a 5-minute massage was as effective as a 2 1/2 minute or a 10-minute massage.

Oleson and Flocco (1993) used a randomized controlled study to test the effectiveness of ear, hand and foot reflexology for treating premenstrual (PMS) symptoms. The treatment group showed a significant reduction in PMS symptoms compared to the placebo reflexology group.

Uses

The following conditions have been treated with reflexology: anemia, arthritis, back problems, carpal tunnel syndrome, constipation, gout, hay fever, high blood pressure, Meniere's Disease, motion sickness, PMS, stress and thyroid problems (Somerville, 1997).

An advantage of reflexology is that it can be performed at home by the client once the main procedures and areas of treatment are understood. Foot and hand charts are readily available at health food stores. Another advantage of reflexology is that if a foot is sprained, the corresponding area on the hand can be worked.

REFERENCES

Ballegaard S, Noorelunds, & Smith DI. (1996). Cost-benefit of combined use of acupuncture Shiatsu and lifestyle adjustment for treatment of patients with severe angina pectoris. *Acupunct Electro Ther Res* 21(3–4):187–197.

Bauer WC, & Dracup KA. (1987). Physiologic effects of back massage in patients with acute myocardial infarction. *Focus on Critical Care Nursing* 14(6):42–46.

Berkson D. (1977). *The Foot Book: Healing the Body Through Reflexology*. New York: Harper and Row.

Chow AE. (1998). Treatment of postoperative nausea and vomiting by acupressure. *Br J Anesthes* 81(1):102.

Corley MC, Ferriter J, Zeh J, & Gifford C. (1995). Physiological and psychological effects of back rubs. *Applied Nursing Research* 8:39–43.

Downing G. (1972). *The Massage Book*. New York: Random House.

Fan Cf, Tanhiu E, Joshi S, Trivedi S, Hong Y, & Shevde K. (1997). Acupressure for prevention of postoperative nausea and vomiting. *Anesthes Anal* 84(4):821–825.

Felhendler D, & Lisander B. (1997). Pressure on acupoints decrease postoperative pain. *Clin J Pain* 12(4):326–329.

Field T, Schanberg SM, Scafidei F, Bauer CR, Vega-Lahr N, Garcia R, Nystrom J, & Kuhn CM. (1986). Tactile/kinesthetic stimulation effects on preterm newborns. *Pediatrics* 77(5):654–658.

Field T, Grizzle N, Scafidi F, & Schanberg S. (1996). Massage and relaxation therapies' effects on depressed adolescent mothers. *Adolescence* 31:903–911.

Gordon A, Merenstein JH, D'Amico F, & Hudgens D. (1998). The effects of therapeutic touch on patients with osteoarthritis of the knee. *J Family Practice* 47(4):271–277.

Groer M, Mozingo J, Droppleman P, Davis M, Jolley M, Boynton M, Davis K, & Kay S. (1994). Measures of salivary immunoglobulin A and state anxiety after a nursing back rub. *Applied Nursing Research* 7(1):2–6.

Hale EH. (1986). A study of the relationship between therapeutic touch and the anxiety of hospitalized patients. Unpublished doctoral dissertation, Texas Women's University.

Harrold F. (1992). *The Complete Body Massage: A Hands-On Manual*. New York: Sterling Publishing Co.

Heidt P. (1979). An investigation of the effects of Therapeutic Touch on anxiety in hospitalized patients. Unpublished doctoral dissertation, New York University.

Hyde E. (1989). Acupressure therapy for morning sickness: A controlled clinical trial. *J Nse Midwifery* 34(4):171–178.

Ireland M. (1998). Therapeutic touch with HIV-infected children: A pilot study. *J Assoc Nurses AIDS Care* 9(4):68–77.

Ironson G, Field TM, Scafidi F, Kumar M, Patarca R, Price A, Goncalves A, Hashimoto M, Kumar A, Burman I, Tetenman C, & Fletcher MA. (1996). Massage therapy is associated with enhancement of the immune system's cytotoxic capacity. *International Journal of Neuroscience* 84:205–218.

Knaster M. (1984). Massage: The roots of women's healing. In K Weiss (Ed.), *Women's Health Care: A Guide to Alternatives*. Reston, VA: Reston Publishing Co.

Koenig S. (1981). Touch for health. In E Bauman (Ed.), *The Holistic Health Life Book* (pp. 44–51). Berkeley, CA: And/Or Press.

Kramer NA. (1990). A comparison of Therapeutic Touch and Casual Touch in stress reduction in hospitalized children. *Ped Nsg* 16(5):483–485.

Krieger D. (1993). *Accepting Your Power to Heal. The Personal Practice of Therapeutic Touch*. Santa Fe, NM: Bear & Company.

Longworth JC. (1982). Psychophysiological effects of slow back massage in normotensive females. *Advances in Nursing Science* 4(4):44–61.

Lowe C & Nechas J. (1983). *Whole Body Healing*. Emmous, PA: Rodale Press, pp. 508–552.

Meehan JC. (1985). The effect of therapeutic touch on the experience of acute pain in postoperative patients. Doctoral dissertation, New York University.

Meek SS. (1993). Effects of slow back massage on relaxation in hospice patients. *Image: Journal of Nursing Scholarship* 25:17–21.

Nickel D. (1984). *Acupressure for Athletes*. Santa Monica, CA: Health AcuPress.

Oleson T, & Flocco W. (1993). Randomized controlled study of premenstrual symptoms treated with ear, hand and foot reflexology. *Obstet & Gynecol* 82(6):906–911.

Patterson A. (1984). Acupressure for women's health. In K. Weiss (Ed.), *Women's Health Care: A Guide to Alternatives* (pp. 270–283). Reston, VA: Reston Publishing Co.

Quinn J. (1982). An investigation of the effects of therapeutic touch done without physical contact on state anxiety of hospitalized patients. Unpublished doctoral dissertation, New York University.

Rice R. (1975). Premature infants respond to sensory stimulation. *APA Monitor* 6(11):8–9.

Robinson N, & Dirnfeld F. (1967). The ionized state of the atmosphere as a function of the meterological elements and the various sources of ions. *Internatl J Brometerol* 11(11):279–288.

Schachner L, Field T, Hernandez-Reif M, Duarte AM, & Krasnegor J. (1998). Atopic dermatitis symptoms decreased in children following massage therapy. *Pediatr Dermatol* 15(5):390–395.

Schneider V. (1979). *Infant Massage*. 2nd ed. Aurora, CO: Vimala Schneider.

Serizawa K. (1972). *Massage the Oriental Method*. Elmsford, NY: Japanese Publications, Inc.

Simington JA, & Laing GGP. (1993). Effects of therapeutic touch on anxiety in institutionalized elderly. *Clinical Nursing Research* 2:438–450.

Snyder M, Egan EC, & Burns KR. (1995). Efficacy of hand massage in decreasing agitation behaviors associated with care activities in persons with dementia. *Geriatric Nursing* 16(2):60– 63.

Snyder M, & Cheng WY. (1998). Massage. In MR Snyder and R Lindquist (Eds.), *Complementary/Alternative Therapies in Nursing*. New York: Springer Publishing Company.

Somerville R. (1997). *The Alternative Advisor*. Richmond, VA: Time-Life Books.

Sunshine W, Field TM, Schanberg S, Quintino O, Kilmer T, Fierro K, Burman I, Hashimoto M, McBride C, & Henteleff T. (1996). Massage therapy and transcutaneous electrical stimulation effects on fibromyalgia. *Journal of Clinical Rheumatology* 2:18–22.

Tappan F. (1984). Massage, reflexology and woman. In K Weiss (Ed.), *Women's Health Care: A Guide to the Alternatives* (pp. 258–269). Reston, VA: Reston Publishing Co.

Turner JG, Clark AJ, Gauthier Dk, & Williams M. (1998). The effect of therapeutic touch on pain and anxiety in burn patients. *J Advanced Nursing* 28(1):10–20.

Wirth DP. (1990). The effect of non-contact therapeutic touch on the healing of full dermal thickness wounds. *Subtle Energies* 1(1):1–20.

Wirth DP. (1993). Full thickness dermal wounds treated with non-contact therapeutic touch: A replication and extension. *Complementary Ther Med* 1:127–132.

Zeidenstein L. (1998). Alternative therapies for nausea and vomiting of pregnancy. *J Nse Midwifery* 43(5):393–393.

D

Therapeutic Activities

26

ART PRODUCTION AND RITUAL

Art is one of the oldest means of communication. Through it, inner thoughts and feelings are expressed. Often these feelings are not conscious. Once projected out onto paper or some other media, feelings can be discussed and healing can occur.

When using art productions/rituals, it is not important that the client use artistically "correct" colors or forms. What is important is that the process is liberating and healing.

Art productions have been used as a healing technique for a full range of human issues and conditions including physical illness, depression, relationship conflicts, divorce, death of a loved one, career crisis, creative blocks, and life "failures" (Capacchione, 1990).

By focusing on the physical symptoms the body presents them with, clients can receive a message about the meaning of the symptom. Pain might mean: "Help, I need to rest," or "Nobody cares about me," or something else. The client is the expert in the meaning of his or her pain. Focusing on the symptom through artwork allows the unconscious to speak. Emotions that have been stuffed into a body part begin to loosen and flow out. Beliefs about life reveal themselves and clients learn to trust their inner wisdom about what the symptom is communicating (Capacchione, 1990).

GOALS FOR ART/RITUAL

Some goals for art production and/or ritual are:

1. Tap inner resources and make meaningful, healing pictures.
2. Find the roots of stress pain and disease.
3. Change beliefs that limit health and well-being.
4. Discover the therapeutic power of creative expression.

USING ART AS ASSESSMENT

A dramatic way for clients to self-assess their level of wellness is through drawing. During this exercise, clients give voice to the their physical sensations. Many learn the unconscious psychological roots for pain or discomfort or unmet needs.

Directions for using this assessment with clients follow (Capacchione, 1990).

1. Close your eyes and get into a comfortable position.
2. Follow the rhythm of the breath as it slows and deepens, nourishing and relaxing you.
3. Start in your left foot and travel through every inch of your body, your toes, heel, top of foot, low leg, thigh and hip, listening to all your physical sensations: comfort, pain, discomfort, cool, hot, empty, wet, dry, tight, loose, and so forth. Go down to your right foot and travel up to your hip in the same manner, noting any physical sensations.
4. Move up your pelvis, front and back, inside and out, your abdominal area, your back and chest.
5. Move up your fingers, hand, and left arm. Repeat on your right side.
6. Focus on your throat and neck, moving through your jaw and face, paying attention to your cheeks, eyes, ears, forehead, scalp, and hair.
7. End at a still point in the center of your head.
8. Using the opposite hand from which you write with, draw your body and the places you felt sensations, using colors that signify specific feelings.
9. Write a dialogue with each of your symptoms or entire mind/body/spirit, using your writing hand to ask the questions and your hand to write the answers.

ART INTERVENTIONS FOR SPECIFIC ISSUES

Drawing taps into inner feelings and beliefs. Drawing with the nondominant hand, the one not used to write with, is believed to tap into the creative, holistic right brain and can often gain access to more fundamental issues.

When working with art production or rituals, it is important to allow individuals to express their feelings about their productions. The practitioner takes care not to analyze or ask specific questions about the productions. It is more helpful to say, "Tell me about your drawing," or "What's going on in this picture," to help facilitate communication.

Abuse

Individuals who have been abused do not feel safe. Creating a safe place can be an important intervention. Use the directions that follow to assist clients to create a safe place.

1. Using your nondominant hand, draw a picture of a place that feels safe to you.
2. Display your drawing in a place you will look at frequently.
3. Draw comfort and solace from your picture.

AIDS or Other Terminal Illnesses

Anger is a powerful and potentially destructive emotion, especially for those diagnosed with AIDS. Through art production, anger can be openly expressed and visibly contained in the media. Safety is enhanced by the boundaries of the paper or other media. The following exercise can be used to assist clients to deal with anger.

1. Think about the situations that have resulted in you feeling angry since you were diagnosed with AIDS.
2. Choose collage pictures or draw symbols or images that express your anger (Landgarten & Lubbers, 1991).

Hope can sustain clients through life-threatening situations. Art can enhance hope. Use the exercise that follows to help clients feel hopeful.

1. Think about things that help you feel better.
2. Draw or choose collage pictures that illustrate those things.

Back Pain

The back supports the rest of the body. As such, it is a metaphor for lack of support. Ask the client who complains of back pain to (1) really listen to the pain and what it is saying; (2) draw pictures of the pain; (3) have a dialogue with the back pain and draw pictures of what is said.

Eating Disorders

Individuals with eating disorders have acted out their conflicts about control and autonomy in the arena of food. A primary focus is to assist them to refocus their energy on ways to gain healthy control and autonomy. Using art materials provides an opportunity for learning new skills of positive self-expansion through the manipulation of media. Early experiences of failure in attempting to communicate feelings often leads to difficulty in recognizing and expressing internal feeling states (Landgarten & Lubbers, 1991).

Use the following exercise to assist individuals with eating disorders to get in touch with their feelings and express them in a self-expansive way.

1. Depict feelings you have had recently in the form of a feeling chart.
2. For each feeling, draw a symbol that has meaning for you.

Individuals with eating disorders feel controlled by one or both parents. Art can be used to help identify these feelings and suggest healthy ways of handling feeling controlled. Use the directions that follow to help with family dynamic issues.

1. Draw a picture of your family.
2. Show the relationships between you and each family member.
3. Use words, symbols, and pictures to dramatize the feelings each family member has for you.
4. Now draw a picture of your ideal family, including actions you can take to feel more comfortable in your family.

Individuals with eating disorders often conceptualize their bodies in a mechanistic or separate fashion. They find it difficult to be realistic about weight and their weight, are often perfectionistic, and have difficulty with their sexual/sensual side. Use the following directions for these issues.

1. Draw a picture of yourself moving for the sake of pleasure.
2. Immerse yourself in that picture, feeling how good it feels to move and feel pleasure.
3. Display the picture you created somewhere where you will view it frequently and obtain pleasure from viewing it.

Individuals with eating disorders are often enmeshed in their family dynamics. Individuation is a primary goal. Use the following exercise to assist in this process.

1. Depict a problem you expect to encounter in the next week.
2. Draw at least two ways you plan to resolve the problem.
3. Congratulate yourself for solving the problem by writing encouraging words on the drawing

Eye Problems

A metaphor for eye problems is that the person "does not want to see" something in his life. Provide drawing materials and ask the client to start drawing himself and his own needs more truthfully and to avoid blaming others for his problems.

Health, General

The body begins to react after carrying around negative pictures of disease, lack of support, dismal life situations, etc. One way to begin to change those negative internal pictures is to draw positive, health-enhancing pictures.

Use the following directions to assist clients to draw health-enhancing pictures of their bodies (Capacchione, 1990).

1. Using your nondominant hand, create a picture of your body as you would like it to feel and be.
2. As you draw, experience feelings of perfect health and vitality.
3. Write words around the picture, detailing your feelings.
4. Ask clients to display their "Pictures of Health" somewhere where they can look at it daily and draw strength and energy from it.

Another health-enhancing tool is the *mandala*, which means "magic circle" in Sanskrit. Use the following directions to help clients create a health-enhancing mandala.

1. Create a circular design in the middle of a page.
2. Radiating out from the center, create up to 8 spokes. Label the pieces of the pie that are created, e.g., body, work, health, relationships, personal growth, spirituality, creativity, leisure.
3. Fill in each piece of the pie with health-enhancing pictures, symbols and/ or words that portray its label.

Nausea

Painting can help shift the focus from mental or physical pain by filling the eye and mind with color and line. Diaz (1992) described a woman who suffered from nausea due to chemotherapy. She found that sitting with a circle in front of her and focusing on the circular design and patterns helped eliminate nausea.

Stress Reduction

Use the following directions to assist clients to reduce stress.

1. Draw a diagram or symbolic picture of the stressful situation based on the following statements:

   A. Ask yourself, what does the situation look like?
   B. Ask yourself, what does the situation feel like?
   C. Create a graphic metaphor that shows your experience of the situation: trapped, overwhelmed, angry, powerless, attacked, etc. Use boxes, mountains, animals, large people, and weapons to depict your feelings.

REFERENCES

Capacchione L. (1990). *The Picture of Health, Healing Your Life with Art.* Santa Monica, CA: Hay House.

Diaz A. (1992). *Freeing the Creative Spirit, Drawing on the Power of Art to Tap the Magic & Wisdom Within.* New York: HarperCollins.

Landgarten HB, & Lubbers D. (1991). *Adult Art Psychotherapy, Issues and Applications.* New York: Brunner/Mazel.

27

JOURNAL WRITING

A journal is a book of dated writings. It can contain the day's events, the writer's feelings, dreams, dialogues, or fantasies. The journal is a tool for recording the process of a life, but journal entries also integrate musculoskeletal processes with memory, and sensory systems, to promote harmony and wholeness (Snyder, 1998). Journaling is a new teaching technique that provides the opportunity for learners to reflect on and analyze their life experiences (Mayo, 1996). Through the journaling process, clients can learn to identify thoughts, feelings, and behavior patterns, as well as solve problems. Because the record is permanent, clients can return to passages again and again to glean new responses to a pattern. While thought patterns often become repetitive and memory fades, a journal preserves the essence of an experience. Working with a journal can also assist clients to think logically and in a goal-oriented manner. Also, while writing or talking to a good listener produces comparable effects (Donnelly & Murray, 1991; Esterling, Antoni, Fletch, Margulies, & Schneiderman, 1994; Segal & Murray, 1994), it is not always easy to find a suitable ear.

Progoff (1975) developed an Intensive Journal method for helping individuals move through uncertain times of transition. The method helps participants to identify stoppages, readjustments, or difficult decisions and restructure life goals. Some of the areas Progoff used are: Steppingstone Periods; Intersections: Roads Taken and Not Taken; Reconstructing an Autobiography; Dialogue, with Persons; Dialogue with Works; Dialogue with the Body; Dialogue with Events, Situations and Circumstances; Working with Dreams; Dialogue with Society; Inner Wisdom Dialogue, and the Open Moment.

Baldwin (1977) says the main use of the journal process is to promote self-understanding. Often, clients have a clear sense that something is wrong in their lives, but they are unable to identify what that something is. Journal writing can help to focus on a portion of life experience and uncover major concerns.

RESEARCH BASE FOR JOURNAL WRITING

Pennebaker and his colleagues used writing as a healing tool. Their work is based on research showing that inhibiting strong feelings gradually undermines the body's defenses. Like other stressors, it can inhibit the immune, cardiovascular, and nervous systems. Confession in writing can neutralize the effects of inhibition (Pennebaker, 1997). Davison (1999) described the use of therapeutic writing as a method for enhancing the immune function.

The research basis for written disclosure was developed and investigated by Pennebaker in the early 1980s. He witnessed the positive physiological and psychological effects of criminal confessions and reasoned that many individuals with no criminal history might have events in their histories that were difficult to discuss with others, but might be negatively affecting their health status because of the stress associated with inhibiting confession. Pennebaker reasoned that if these individuals wrote about traumatic events or upsetting issues, they might experience improvement in their health and might be able to do so without the social risks (awkwardness, judgment, or recrimination) associated with confiding in another person (Davison, 1999).

To test the hypothesis, Pennebaker and Beall (1986) randomly assigned 80 undergraduates to either treatment (write about their deepest thoughts and feelings surrounding their most upsetting event or issue ever faced), or control (write about a trivial, nonemotional topic). A third group was asked to write about only their feelings surrounding the topic. In the 3-month follow-up, the treatment group made significantly fewer health center visits for illness than the other two groups.

In 1988, Pennebaker and colleagues measured the immune system effects of emotional disclosure. Blood samples were taken before and after writing in two groups: those who wrote about either upsetting events or trivial topics. Those writing about upsetting topics showed better responses to a number of antigenic challenges than those who wrote about trivial topics.

A later study (Petrie et al., 1995) assessed the impact of disclosure on *in vivo* measures of immune function—response to Hepatitis B vaccination series. The group writing about emotionally charged subjects showed higher responses to the series than did the control group, and higher reductions in skin conductance levels (a measure of sympathetic nervous system arousal associated with the stress of information inhibition).

Other portions of the body are also affected by disclosure in writing. Pennebaker and colleagues (1990) found that writing about coming to college was associated with fewer illness visits to physicians and higher grades in the semester after writing.

Spera and colleagues (1994) found that men who had been laid off from their jobs who wrote about that experience felt less depressed and angry almost immediately. Conversely, when individuals are in a positive frame of mine, writing about a distressing situation dampens their mood.

Runions (1984) also mentioned using journal writing to obtain therapeutic results. The mother of a seriously ill adolescent was asked by the author to keep a journal and to evaluate the results. The client found that journaling enhanced her coping skills.

Hall (1990) reported on the use of journaling with high school students. Results included an enhanced ability to accept their potentialities and manage conflict.

Johnson and Kelly (1990) reported using a journal to help individuals diagnosed with cancer to help them gain insight into their lives and the cancer experience.

USES OF JOURNALING

Disclosure through writing can be used to help individuals faced with chronic or life-threatening illnesses to process and understand the role of their condition in their lives. This type of writing can also assist writers to develop conceptions of the cause and impact of the condition.

Journaling also provides a context for change. In order for change to occur, individuals must prepare interior acceptance for change and provide internal and external support systems for making change. Journal work can provide both (Baldwin, 1977).

Specific individuals who may benefit from journal writing include those faced with:

1. heart disease (Tavris, 1989).
2. cancer (Esterling et al., 1994).
3. pain, especially backache and headache (Jamner & Schwartz, 1986; Traue & Pennebaker, 1993).
4. downsizing (Spera, Buhrfeind, & Pennebaker, 1994).
5. childhood asthma (Florin et al., 1993).
6. secrets they fear disclosing, e.g., gay men who inhibit telling others about their homosexual status (Cole, Kemeny, Taylor, & Visscher, 1996a and 1996b).
7. depression (Baldwin, 1977).
8. eating disorders (Baldwin, 1977).
9. death or separation from important others (Baldwin, 1977).

Specific directions for using journal writing with clients include asking clients to:

1. Purchase a journal that has meaning for them. The size, color, number of pages, etc. is dependent on what feels right for the client.
2. Choose a writing implement that allows for free-flowing writing.
3. Sit in a quiet place for a few moments in stillness. Let the breathing become slow and deep.
4. Begin writing by saying to themselves: "I'm thinking about _____" (topic), remembering journaling is not writing down thoughts, but rather allowing deeper thoughts and feelings to rise up from inside themselves. This free-flowing writing pays no attention to the structure of what is written.
5. Trust the process of resonance that occurs as the flow of energy produces words.

6. Begin a journal entry entitled "Expectations of myself" and use the information to remember how expectations can sabotage growth.
7. Constantly question: What am I leaving out of this entry? Do I forgive myself and others for past experiences? What family myths am I still adhering to that prevent me from being totally honest in my journaling?
8. Always let the original writing stand, but go back frequently to re-read entries and add to them, after the original entry, as new ideas and memories surface.

Some client assignments that may prove helpful are (Baldwin, 1977; Progoff, 1975):

1. Examine your feelings about privacy and sharing and how they relate to your journal. (Clients must first work through any fears of others reading their work before they can be open and honest. Without this step, they may find themselves censoring what they write.)
2. Go back and write about those parts of yourself that got lost along the way.
3. Write positive statements about your behavior and then read them back to enhance your confidence.
4. Allow yourself to imagine what life would have been like had you made decisions opposite from what you made. Go down roads not taken and write down what you see and observe.
5. Write about your ideal day, then find a way to make it happen.
6. What leftover experiences from previous situations are influencing the way I feel and behave now?
7. Explore how your feelings about your body were developed by asking: How did my parents feel about their bodies? What were my family rules for touching, nudity, sex and affection? Were there traumatic instances connected to my early sexual awareness and how have I worked to resolve them? What am I doing to get positive touch today?
8. Gain experience in dealing with grief and loss by writing responses to the following questions: How will I deal with the loss(es) I am facing? Who and what do I need to say goodbye to and how will I accomplish this?
9. Write about how a physical affliction affects your life, how you are changing because of the affliction, and what plans you have for making your life more positive.
10. Choose a relationship you wish to enhance. Write to the relationship as if it were a person, noting significant events and their effects and offering a plan for resolving unresolved parts of the relationship.
11. Choose a person you believe to be wise. Have an imaginary dialogue with that person about a problem in your life. Write down any ideas you have after the dialogue that can be incorporated into your daily regime.

REFERENCES

Baldwin C. (1977). *One to One, Self-Understanding Through Journal Writing.* Philadelphia, PA: J.B. Lippincott and Company.

Cole SW, Kemeny ME, Taylor SE, & Visscher BR. (1996a). Accelerated course of human immunodeficiency virus infection in gay men who conceal their homosexual identity. *Psychosom Med* 58:219–231.

Cole SW, Kemeny ME, Taylor SE, & Visscher BR. (1996b). Elevated physical health risk among gay men who conceal their homosexual identity. *Health Psychology* 15:243–251.

Davison KP. (1999). Therapeutic writing and the immune function. In CC Clark (Ed.), *The Encyclopedia of Complementary Health Practice.* New York: Springer Publishing Company.

Donnelly DA, & Murray EJ. (1991). Cognitive and emotional changes in written essays and therapy interviews. *Journal of Social and Clinical Psychology* 10:334–350.

Esterling BA, Antoni MH, Fletch MA, Margulies S, & Schneiderman N. (1994). Emotional disclosure through writing or speaking modulates latent Epstein-Barr virus reactivation. *Journal of Consulting and Clinical Psychology* 62:130–140.

Hall EG. (1990). Strategies for using journal writing in counseling gifted students. *The Gifted Child Today* 13(4):2–6.

Florin I, Fiegenbaum W, Hermanns J, Winter H, Schobinger R, & Jenkins M. (1993). Emotional expressiveness, psychophysiological reactivity and mother-child intereaction with asthmatic children. In H Traue and JW Pennebaker (Eds.), *Emotion, Inhibition and Health* (pp. 179–196). Seattle: Hogrefe & Huber.

Jamner LD & Schwartz GE. (1986). Self-deception predicts self-report and endurance of pain. *Psychosom Med* 48:211–223.

Jamner LD, Shapiro D, Hui KK, & Oakley ME. (1993). Hostility and differences between clinic, self-determined, and ambulatory blood pressure. *Psychosom Med* 55:203–211.

Johnson JB, & Kelly AW. (1990). A multifaceted rehabilitation program for women with cancer. *Oncology Nursing Forum* 17:691–695.

Mayo K. (1996). Social responsibility in nursing education. *Journal of Holistic Nursing* 14:24–32.

Pennebaker JW, & Beall SK. (1986). Confronting a traumatic event: Toward an understanding of inhibition and disease. *Journal of Abnormal Psychology* 95:274–281.

Pennebaker JW, Kiecolt-Glaser J, & Glaser R. (1988). Disclosure of traumas and immune function: Health implications for psychotherapy. *Journal of Clinical and Consulting Psychology* 63:787–792.

Pennebaker JW, Colder M, & Sharp L. (1990). Accelerating the coping process. *Journal of Personality and Social Psychology* 58:528–537.

Pennebaker JW. (1997). *Opening Up, The Healing Power of Expressing Emotions.* New York: Guilford Press.

Petrie KJ, Boothe RJ, Pennebaker JW, Davison KP, & Thomas M. (1995). Disclosure of trauma and immune response to Hepatitis B vaccination program. *Journal of Consult & Clin Psychol* 63:787–792.

Progoff I. (1975). *At A Journal Workshop, The Basic Text and Guide for Using the Intensive Journal.* New York: Dialogue House Library.

Runions J. (1984). The diary: A self-directed approach to coping with stress. *Canadian Nurse* 80(5):24–28.

Segal DL, & Murray EJ. (1994). Emotional processing in cognitive therapy and vocal expression of feeling. *Journal of Social and Clinical Psychology* 13:189–206.

Snyder M. (1998). Journal Writing. In M. Snyder and R. Lindquist (Eds.), *Complementary/Alternative Therapies in Nursing*. New York: Springer Publishing Company.

Spera SP, Buhrfeind ED, & Pennebaker JW. (1994). Expressive writing and coping with job loss. *Academy of Management Journal* 37:722–733.

Surbeck E, Han EP, & Moyer JE. (1991). Assessing reflective response in journals. *Educational Leadership* 48(6):25–27.

Tavris C. (1989). *Anger: The Misunderstood Emotion*. New York: Simon & Schuster.

Traue HC, & Pennebaker JW. (1993). *Emotion, Inhibition, and Health*. Seattle: Hogrefe & Huber.

28

SOUND/MUSIC THERAPY

Theoretical quantum physics postulates that matter could not exist without consciousness to perceive it. As a result, everything in the universe has an inherent probability-vibrational pattern (Bell, 1987). Sound/Music therapy is based on the theory that when musical vibrations are in tune with human vibratory patterns, a profound healing effect occurs throughout the body (Brewer, 1998).

Just as quantum physics forces the believer to cross the line between truth and myth (Drohan, 1998), a resonance of some kind, a music, puts the practitioner in "tune" with the universe of the client, affecting a change. Drohan (1998) consciously tries to hear her own music when working with clients, sensing vibrational patterns, and providing "restorative patterns" by helping to choose music with the client that can make material changes in his or her wellness.

RESEARCH BASE

The health status of individuals may be displayed in the sound of their voice. Holl (1996) investigated whether health problems could be displayed in voice patterns. The study was based on the Bio-Acoustic energy theory that the body is composed of dense energy patterns. Bio-Acoustics means "life sounds" and involves the study of frequencies emanating from living organisms. When individuals are having positive reactions to specific notes, they will comment that they like the sound. Conversely, when negative reactions occur, the heart rate will significantly increase or decrease, oxygen saturation will decrease, dizziness or restlessness may result, and individuals may comment that they feel relieved when the sound is turned off.

Nonharmonious notes are emanated when individuals are dis-eased. Holl (1996) used a computer program to identify nonharmonious notes in a convenience sample of 26 residents of a nursing home. Residents with osteoarthritis and osteoporosis had notes E and G distressed significantly more than participants without these bone diseases. Note: the vibratory rate of calcium (note E) and magnesium (note G) in distress are the notes in distress for the individuals suffering from osteoporosis.

Individuals with chronic fatigue are likely to have notes F and F ♯ in distress, or their reciprocals, notes B and C, depending on their brain dominance. Residents with Parkinson's disease, who usually have a dopamine deficiency, frequently have note D ♯ in distress. Note: The molecular weight for dopamine is similar to the numeric frequency of D ♯ (Edwards, 1994).

A special kind of "brain music" was used in one study to treat insomnia. Fifty-eight individuals with insomnia were randomly assigned to either an experimental group (who listened to brain music developed by transforming their EEGs into music), or a placebo group (who listened to the brain music of another person). All participants listened to the resulting audio cassettes before going to sleep. Clinical, questionnaire, electrophysical (both polysomnographic and electroen-cephalographic) measures were used before and after 15-day treatment courses. Both subjective and objective measures showed that for more than 80% of the participants there was a positive effect from listening to their own brain music. No side effects or complications were found.

Chian (1998) reported on the effectiveness of music therapy on relaxation and anxiety for participants receiving ventilatory assistance. Fifty-four alert and nonsedated individuals from intensive care units receiving mechanical ventilation were randomized to either a 30-minute music treatment or a rest period. State anxiety, heart rate, and respiratory rate measures were obtained every 5 minutes for 30 minutes. A single music therapy session was effective in significantly decreasing anxiety and promoting relaxation, as indicated by decreases in heart and respiratory rate in individuals receiving ventilatory assistance.

Pacchetti and colleagues (1998) reported on the effect of music therapy on Parkinson's disease (PD). Sixteen individuals diagnosed with PD took part in 13 weekly sessions of music therapy. Every two weeks at the beginning and end of each session, participants were evaluated by a neurologist for PD severity. Emotional functions were evaluated with Happiness Measures and quality of life was assessed using the Parkinson's Disease Quality of Life Questionnaire. There was a significant improvement in motor function after every session. Quality of life and emotional functions also improved.

Clark and colleagues (1998) studied the use of music to decrease aggressive behaviors in individuals with dementia. Eighteen elders were randomly assigned to either treatment (favorite music played during bath) or control (no music). Yelling, abusive language, hitting, verbal resistance, and physical resistance occurred significantly less often when music was played.

Other research on the use of music as a therapeutic tool include: decreasing anxiety (Klein & Winkelstein, 1996; Barnason, Zimmerman, & Nieveen, 1995); reducing agitation during meals (Goddaer & Abraham, 1994); pain management (Good, 1995); sleep disturbances (Mornhinweg & Voignier, 1995); death and dying (Schroeder-Sheker, 1994); decreasing stress and enhancing relaxation (Chlan, 1995); reducing high arousal states in neonates (Kaminski & Hall, 1996); and, improving psychotic symptoms (Lee, Yeh, & Lie, 1993).

THERAPEUTIC USES OF MUSIC/SOUND

Table 28.1 provides a list of the specific effects of music as a therapeutic modality. Specific kinds of music are also identified.

Table 28.1 Possible Therapeutic Uses of Music/Sound

Effect	Type of Music Suggested
Mask unpleasant sounds; can be used during dental procedures or other noisy health care situations to dispel the turmoil created by the sounds and vibrations of health care equipment and instruments	Quiet baroque; humming.*
Slow down and equalize brain waves, shifting the brain to alpha waves, providing calming and heightened awareness: use for anxiety, conflict, Alzheimer's, Parkinson's	10–15 minutes of Mozart, Bach, baroque, or New Age music; Chopin's nocturnes to the Sunset or Evening; Ragas of classical Indian music.
Evoke emotion in individuals not able to express their feelings, e.g., grief	Tchaikovsky and Rachmaninoff; Stravinsky's "The Rite of Spring"; Rodrigo's "Concierto Aranjuez."
Affect heartbeat	The faster the music, the faster the heart will beat; avoid rock music; it has negative effects on the heart; try some Mozart or reading aloud from Shakespeare (iambic pentameter closely parallels the heart beating at 65–75 beats a minute).
Lower blood pressure	Don Campbell's "Essence: Crystal Meditations;" Indian ragas; Daniel Kobialka's "Timeless Lullaby" (excessive noise can raise the blood pressure by up to 10 percent).
Reduce muscle tension and improves body movement and coordination	3–4 minutes of Spanish guitar music for stretching and yoga; active movement to "Riverdance"; cool down to Mozart symphony or string quartet.
Affect body temperature	Warm, friendly music with a strong beat, warms; detached, abstract music, cools.
Increase endorphin levels and lessen pain	Movie soundtracks, religious music, marching bands, or drumming ensembles.
Regulate stress-related hormones	Beethoven sonatas.

(continued)

Table 28.1 *(continued)*

Effect	Type of Music Suggested
Boost immune function	Mozart; music of the client's choice including New Age selections, mild jazz, Mozart, and Ravel.
Change perception of space	Mozart's chamber music or Halpern's "Spectrum Suite" is relaxing and gives a sense of not being confined.
Change perception of time	To slow down: highly romantic or New Age; To speed up: marching music; To order behavior: classical and baroque music.
Energize or influence	Drums.
Enhance and strengthen memory	Studying: Mozart or Vivaldi in the background; Memorizing: Baroque music; Enhance concentration: Haydn and Mozart.
Boost productivity	Light classical music.
Enhance romance and sexuality	"Moonlight Sonata," "Out of Africa" soundtrack; Schubert, Schumann, Tchaikovsky, Chopin, or Liszt.
Boost creativity	Debussy, Faure, or Ravel.
Create group identity	Seniors drumming to Lawrence Welk or other music of their generation; Young people jam to Gloria Estefan, Hootie and the Blowfish; Encourage improvisation on a variety of percussion instruments to teach listening and cooperation.
Stimulate digestion	Eat faster and more: rock music; Eat slower and less: classical music.
Foster endurance	"I've Been Working on the Railroad"; Synchronized high-performance music tapes.
Create safety and well-being	The popular music of the client's era; slower baroque music: Bach, Handel, Vivaldi, Corelli.
Reduce inappropriate behavior in youngsters	Beatles.
Inspire	Jazz, the blues, Dixieland, soul, calypso, reggae.
Soothe while awakening	Samba.
Increase respiration and heartbeat, get the body moving	Salsa, rhumba, maranga, macarena.

Table 28.1 *(continued)*

Effect	Type of Music Suggested
Release the tensions of adolescence	Punk, heavy metal, and other popular music.
Cleanse emotions	Babble in nonsense syllables to an interested listener who does not comment about something that is stressing.
Restore voice	Hum, especially "m."
Reduce reading difficulties	Read aloud to a slow second movement of a baroque concerto by Bach or Handel.
Learn a language	Play classical or folk music in the background to anchor instruction.
Relieve pain	Make an "ah" or "ou" sound and visualize pain being released through the voice; listen to gospel music.
Keep alert	High "ee" voice sound for 3–5 minutes.
Stimulate immune system	Hum lullabies.
Stir the growth of plants	Bach and Indian music.
Aid language-impaired (stroke suffers, accident victims, aphasics) who cannot understand the plainly spoken word	Rap music.
Build self-confidence	Make vowel sounds out loud and create sounds that represent joy and peace.
Heal after surgery	Listen to favorite music during surgery or Helen Bonny's "Music Rx" tapes.
Reduce nasal congestion	Hum, make "Ah" sounds or make an "nggg" sound in the back of the throat.
Control headaches	Make "Ouuu" sounds and listen to them vibrate throughout the head; listen to Mozart's *Symphony No. 39 in E flat* (KV.543) and piano concerto *No. 12 in A Major* (K. 414).
Reduce menopausal symptoms	Make vowel sounds, focusing on the vibrations in the pelvic area.
Reduce gait disorders	Using a cassette headphone, step on the first beat, the first and third beat, or every eighth beat to "Stars and Stripes Forever," "Seventy-Six Trombones," or "Semper Fidelis."
Assist labor and delivery	Tone "Ah" and "Oh" through contractions, letting the sound align the body, and keep the mother focused.

(continued)

Table 28.1   *(continued)*

Effect	Type of Music Suggested
Premature infants	Play or sing to them: "You Are My Sunshine," or Brahm's "Lullaby."
Psychotic auditory hallucinations	Hum the "Mmm" sound.

Sources: Richard Del Maestro (1994). Music and healing. *Atlantis, the Imagery Newsletter* (December):1–2,4; Don Campbell (1997). New York: Avon Books; Deepak Chopra (1997). Ayurveda: The sounds of music. *Infinite Possibilities* 2(1):3.

REFERENCES

Barnason S, Zimmerman L, & Nieveen J. (1995). The effects of music interventions on anxiety in the patient after coronary artery bypass grafting. *Heart & Lung: Journal of Critical Care* 24(2):124–132.

Bell J. (1987). *Speakable and Unspeakable in Quantum Mechanics*. Cambridge, England: Cambridge University Press.

Brewer JF. (1998). Healing sounds. *Complement Ther Nurs Midwifery* 4(1):7–12.

Chian L. (1998). Effectiveness of a music therapy intervention on relaxation and anxiety for patients receiving ventilatory assistance. *Heart/Lung* 27(3):169–176.

Chlan I. (1995). Psychophysiologic responses of mechanically ventilated patients to music: A pilot study. *American Journal of Critical Care* 4(3):233–238.

Clark ME, Lipe AW, & Bilbrey BA. (1998). Use of music to decrease aggressive behaviors in people with dementia. *Journal of Gerontol Nursing* 24(7):10–17.

Drohan M. (1998). From myth to reality: How music changes matter. Submitted for publication to *Alternative Health Practitioner: The Journal of Complementary and Natural Care*.

Edwards S. (1994). Signature sound: Research and results. Presented at the Forum II Workshop, Athens, OH.

Goddaer HM, & Abraham IL. (1994). Effects of relaxing music on agitation during meals among nursing home residents with severe cognitive impairment. *Archives of Psychiatric Nursing* 8(3):150–158.

Good M. (1995). A comparison of the effects of jaw relaxation and music on postoperative pain. *Nursing Research* 44(1):52–57.

Holl R. (1996). Health problems displayed in voice patterns. *Alternative Health Practitioner: The Journal of Complementary and Natural Care* 2(3):169–175.

Kaminski J, & Hall W. (1996). The effect of soothing music on neonatal behavioral states in the hospital newborn nursery. *Neonatal Network: Journal of Neonatal Nursing* 15(1):45–54.

Klein S, & Winkelstein M. (1996). Enhancing pediatric health care with music. *Pediatric Health Care* 19(1):74–81.

Lee S, Yeh MY, & Lie TZ. (1993). Effects of music therapy on improving psychotic symptoms and personal interactions of psychotic patients. *Nursing Research (China)* 1(2):145–157.

Mornhinweg G, & Voignier R. (1995). Music for sleep disturbance in the elderly. *Journal of Holistic Nursing* 13(3):248–254.

Pacchetti C, Agileri R, Mancini F, Martignoni E, & Nappi G. (1998). Active music therapy and Parkinson's disease: Methods. *Funct Neurol* 13(1):57–67.

Schroeder-Sheker T. (1994). Music for the dying: A personal account of the new field of music thanatology. *Journal of Holistic Nursing* 12(1):83–99.

APPENDIX: TRAINING PROGRAMS, EDUCATIONAL RESOURCES, AND ORGANIZATIONS

ACUPRESSURE (see also: Chinese Health and Healing, chapter 13)
Acupressure Institute. 1533 Shattuck Avenue, Berkeley, CA 94709. Phone: (510)845-1059.
The Main Central. Jin Shin Jyutsu, Inc., 8719 E. San Alberto, Scottsdale, AZ 85258. Phone: (602)998-9331, Fax: (602)998-9335.

AROMATHERAPY
Aromatherapy Institute of Research. P.O. Box 2354, Fair Oaks, CA 95628. Phone: (916)965-7546.
Aromatherapy Seminars. 3384 S. Robertson Place, Los Angeles, CA 90034.
Pacific Institute of Aromatherapy. P.O. Box 606, San Rafael, CA 94915.

AYURVEDA
The American Institute of Vedic Studies. P.O. Box 8357, Santa Fe, NM 87504-8357. Phone: (505)983-9385.
The American School of Ayurvedic Sciences. 10025 N.E. 4th, Bellevue, WA 98004. Phone: (206)453-8022, Fax: (206)451-2670.
The Ayurveda Holistic Center of New York. 82A Bayville Avenue, Bayville, NY 11709. Phone/Fax: (516)628-8200.
Ayurveda Institute. P.O. Box 23445, Albuquerque, NM 87192-1445. Phone: (505)291-9698, Fax: (505)294-7572.
Bastyr University of Natural Health Sciences. 144 N.E. 54th Street, Seattle, WA 98105. Phone (206)523-9585, Fax: (206) 527-4763.

The Center for Mind/Body Medicine. P.O. Box 1048, La Jolla, CA 92038-1048. Phone: (619)794-2425, Fax: (619)794-2440.

College of Maharishi Ayur-Ved. Maharisha International University, 1000 4th Street, DB-1155, Fairfield, IA 52557-1155. Phone: (515)472-7000, Fax: (375)472-1189.

Vedic Sciences Institute. P.O. Box 2537, Jupiter, FL 33468-2537. Phone: (407) 745-2164.

GUIDED IMAGERY

Academy for Guided Imagery. P.O. Box 2070, Mill Valley, CA 94942. Phone: (800)726-2070.

American Institute for Mental Imagery. 351 E. 84th Street, Suite 10D, New York, NY 10028.

Guided Imagery and Music. Music-Centered Psychotherapy, 2801 Buford Highway, Suite 225, Atlanta, GA 30329. Phone: (404)8224.

HEART PROGRAM

Dean Ornish's Opening Your Heart Program. Preventive Medicine Research Medicine Research Institute, 900 Bridgeway, Suite 2, Sausalito, CA 94965. Phone: (415)332-2525.

HERBS

American Botanical Council. P.O. Box 201660, Austin, TX 78720. Phone: (512)331-8868.

American Herb Association. P.O. Box 1673, Nevada City, CA 95959. Phone: (916)265-9552.

Herb Research Foundation. 1007 Pearl Street, Suite 200, Boulder, CO 80302. Phone: (303)449-2265.

National College of Phytotherapy. 120 Aliso S.E., Albuquerque, NM 87108. Phone: (505)265-0795, Fax: (505)232-3522.

HYPNOSIS

American Association of Professional Hypnotherapies. P.O. Box, Boones Mill, VA 24065. Phone: (703)334-3035.

American Psychological Association. Psychological Hypnosis, Division 30, 750 First Street, NE, Washington, DC 20002. Phone: (202)336-5500.

American Society of Clinical Hypnosis. 2200 East Devon Avenue, Suite 291, Des Plaines, IL 60018. Phone: (708)297-3317.

American Academy of Scientific Hypnotherapy. P.O. Box 12041, San Diego, CA 92112. Phone: (619)427-6225.

International Medical and Dental Hypnotherapy Association. 4110 Edgeland, Suite 800, Royal Oaks, MI 48703-2251. Phone: (810)549-5594.

National Society of Hypnotherapists. 2175 NW 86th, Suite 6A, Des Moines, IA 50325. Phone: (515)270-2280.

Society for Clinical and Experimental Hypnosis. 6728 Old McLean Village Drive, McLean, VA 22101-3906. Phone: (703)556-9222.

MASSAGE
American Massage Therapy Association. 820 Davis Street, Suite 100, Evanston, IL 60201. Phone: (847)864-0123, http://www.amtamassage.org.
Center for Human Caring. University of Colorado Health Sciences Center, 4200 E. 9th Avenue, Denver, CO 80262. Phone: (303)270-6157, http://www.uchsc.edu/ctrsinst.chc.

ORIENTAL MEDICINE
American Association of Oriental Medicine. 433 Front Street, Catasauqua, PA 18032. Phone: (610)266-1433, http://www.aaom.org.
American Foundation of Traditional Chinese Medicine. 505 Beach Street, San Francisco, CA 94133. Phone: (415)776-0502.
Oregon College of Oriental Medicine. 10525 S.E. Cherry Blossom Drive, Portland, OR 97216. Phone: (503)253-3443, Fax: (503)253-2701.

REFLEXOLOGY
American Reflexology Certification Board and Information Service. P.O. Box 246654, Sacramento, CA 95824. Phone: (916)455-5381.

STRESS REDUCTION
University of Massachusetts Medical Center. 55 Lake Avenue North, Worchester, MA 01655. Phone: (508) 856-0011, http://www.ummed.edu.

THERAPEUTIC TOUCH
American Holistic Nurses Association. P.O. Box 2130, Flagstaff, AZ 86003-2130, http:www/ahna.org.
College of New Rochelle Graduate School of Nursing. 29 Castle Place, New Rochelle, NY 10805. Phone: 1-800-211-7077.
Nurse Healers Professional Associates, Inc. 1211 Locust Street, Philadelphia, PA 19107. Phone: (215)545-8079, http://www.therapeutic-touch.org.

TOUCH
Wellness Resources. 16741 Gulf Boulevard, N. Redington Beach, FL 33708. Phone: (727) 320-9066, http://home.earthlink.net/~cccwellness.
Caring Touch for the Frail, Elderly, or Dying Client. Barbara Harris, RN, BA, LMT, HNC, 147 Windward Drive, Osprey, FL 34229. Phone: (941)966-6961.

INDEX

Ⓢ *Springer Publishing Company*

Alternative Therapies
Expanding Options in Health Care

Rena J. Gordon, PhD, **Barbara Cable Nienstedt,** DPA,
Wilbert M. Gesler, PhD, Editors

"...an excellent text for understanding the ebb and flow of alternative ther-
apies in the American health system. It can served both as a fine introduc-
tion for the uninitiated to the history and issues surrounding alternative
therapies in the United States, and as a valuable resource for specialists in
the field. The inclusion of regional/geographic approaches is an especially
valuable - and often overlooked - contribution."

-Paul Root Wolpe, PhD
Center for Bioethics, University of Pennsylvania

"This book should be required reading for health care practitioners, particu-
larly physicians and nurses, who intend to be practicing in the next centu-
ry...[It] can be used as an undergraduate or graduate text in an advanced
course on alternative/complementary therapies, or as a reference work to be
used in a variety of courses throughout a variety of curricula..."

-Gloria F. Donnelly, PhD, RN, FAAN
Dean and Professor, School of Nursing,
Allegheny University of the Health Sciences

Contents: Introduction: Alternative Therapies: Why Now? • The
Definitional Dilemma of Alternative Medicine • Politics and the Law:
The Federal Approach to Alternative Medicine: Co-opting, Quack-
busting, or Complementing? • The Power of the State • Paradigms
and Politics: Redux of Homeopathy in American Medicine • The
Changing Medical Marketplace: Marketing Channels for Alternative
Health Care • The Regional Distribution of Alternative Health Care •
Demand for Alternative Therapies: The Case of Childbirth • The
Culture Complex: Social and Cultural Aspects of Alternative Therapies
• Building Medical Systems at the Household Level • Redefining the
Healing Process: Healer-Client Relationships in Alternative Medicine
• Toward Complementary Medicine: Rediscovering Nightingale:
Back to the Future • Biomedical Physicians Practicing Holistic Medi-
cine • Medical Education: Changes and Responses • Alternative
Therapies: Quo Vadis?

1998 296pp. 0-8261-1164-5 hard www.springerpub.com

536 Broadway, New York, NY 10012-3955 • (212) 431-4370 • Fax (212) 941-7842

Springer Publishing Company

A Total Wellness Program for Women Over 30

Comprehensive Manual with Medical Guidelines for Health Care Professionals

Barbara Kass-Annese, RNCNP, MSN, Consultants, **William Parker,** MD, and **Sharon Schnare,** RN, FNP, CNM

"An A to Z comprehensive guide for health care professionals and a significant contribution for the treatment of women."
> –**Marie Lugani**, President and founder of the American Menopause Foundation Inc.

This manual provides a comprehensive wellness program for women in preparation as they age. It blends western conventional medicine with complementary (alternative) health care practices. The total wellness approach includes exercise, nutrition, vitamin and mineral therapy, and stress management as its foundation.

Contents: Acknowledgements • Introduction • From Perimenopause to Postmenopause • Symptoms of the Climacteric • Cardiovascular Disease • Osteoporosis and Other Health Issues • Psychological, Sociological, and Sexual Issues Associated with the Climacteric • A Total Wellness Program for Women • Hormonal and Drug Therapies • Complementary Therapies, Holistic Medicine • Final Remarks • Guidelines for the Care of Women Over 30 • In Closing • Appendix A • Appendix B • Bibliography and Resources • References • Evaluation Form

1997 429pp. 0-8261-1180-7 softcover www.springerpub.com

536 Broadway, New York, NY 10012-3955 • (212) 431-4370 • Fax (212) 941-7842